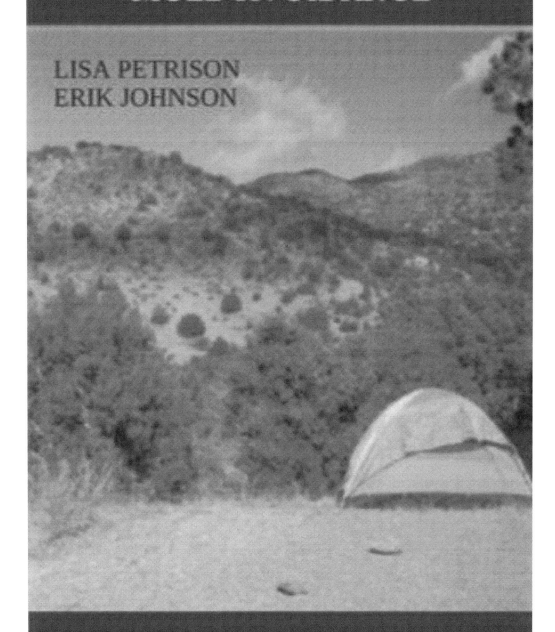

A Beginner's Guide To
MOLD AVOIDANCE

LISA PETRISON
ERIK JOHNSON

Techniques Used by Hundreds of
Chronic Multisystem Illness Sufferers
To Improve Their Health

"A Beginner's Guide to Mold Avoidance: Techniques Used by Hundreds of Chronic Multisystem Illness Sufferers to Improve Their Health"

Text by Lisa Petrison & Erik Johnson.

Photos by Lisa Petrison.

Published by Paradigm Change.

To make comments or ask questions about this book, please contact:

info@paradigmchange.me

For more information about the role of mold toxins in chronic multisystem illness, please visit the Paradigm Change website:

www.paradigmchange.me

More information about mold avoidance from the authors of this book:

www.paradigmchange.me/avoidance/

A list of links related to the information in each chapter of this book:

www.paradigmchange.me/links/

TABLE OF CONTENTS

Part 8 - Social Issues

Chapter 54 - Rebuilding a Life

Chapter 55 - Managing the Responses of Others

Part 9 - Appendices

Appendix 1 - Chronic Multisystem Illnesses

Appendix 2 - Glossary

Appendix 3 - About the Authors

Appendix 4 – Disclaimer & Safety Issues

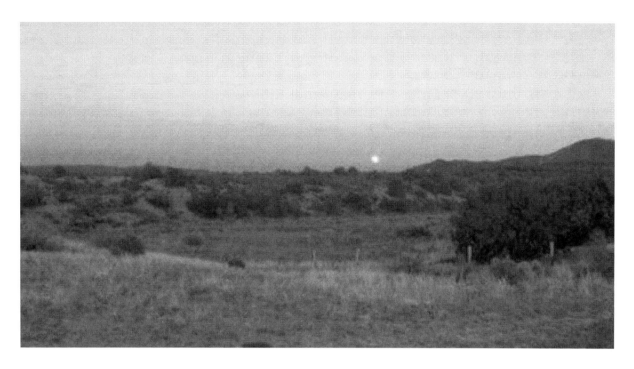

A full moon in northern New Mexico.

Introduction

Disgracefully, many of the sickest people on the planet have been almost wholly ignored by the medical community.

Sufferers of this specific type of illness may experience a wide variety of life-destroying symptoms, including severe cognitive dysfunction, inability to sit or stand, excruciating headaches, extreme noise and light sensitivities, muscle pain, heart dysfunction, immune system abnormalities that allow their bodies to be ravaged by a variety of pathogens, exertion intolerance, seizures, dystonia, wasting, partial paralysis and many others.

Although some sufferers of this disease are able to work with difficulty at least part-time, many are totally disabled for decades.

People with this disease get sick young, usually in their 20's or 30's.

Almost all remain sick permanently. Many die at a relatively young age.

The most severe sufferers spend decades of their lives curled up in darkened silent rooms – unable even to sit up, to tolerate any light or sound, to experience restful sleep, to summon the strength to speak or feed themselves, or to focus on or articulate a thought.

Some specialists have compared the level of debilitation in this population to that experienced by untreated AIDS patients in their last few months of life.

Under the Radar

Traditionally, people with this type of illness have been referred to in the literature as having myalgic encephalomyelitis (ME).

The governments of the US, UK and other countries currently acknowledge this condition only under the much broader illness category that they call "chronic fatigue syndrome."

Some people with this kind of illness self-identify with other disease categories, such as chronic Lyme disease, fibromyalgia, Gulf War illness, multiple chemical sensitivity, toxic mold illness or postural orthostatic tachycardia (POTS).

Regardless of what it is called, this disease has remained under the radar and – considering its prevalence and severity – has continued to be remarkably overlooked.

Treatment Responses

Especially in its most severe form, this disease has proven to be extremely difficult to treat.

Although a few caring physicians have made it their life's work to try to help these severely ill patients, the extent to which they have been able to do so has been very limited.

Virtually all of the individuals with this disease have remained very ill regardless of what medical treatments they have pursued.

Mold Avoidance

The mold avoidance approach described in this book was developed with the goal of helping these extremely ill and stubbornly treatment-resistant individuals.

The underlying premise of the approach presented here is that many or all of these individuals suffer from a severe hyperreactivity to certain kinds of mold toxins.

This approach suggests that insofar as individuals are reacting to very low levels of these mold toxins, decreasing exposures to a level that does not prompt a reaction will allow movement toward wellness to be achieved.

Both of the authors of this book were very sick with this kind of illness for many years and have become mostly recovered as a result of this approach.

During recent years, many other individuals who were very ill with this sort of disease also have experienced major improvements as a result of following this approach.

This book is designed to share the basics of the approach with a broader audience, so that more sufferers can learn about it and decide if it might be worth pursuing.

Because individuals with this type of illness have cognitive issues, the book is written in a simplified style that they may be able to process more easily.

Less Severe Sufferers

This approach was developed specifically for people who are extremely ill and who have not made substantial improvements through any other therapies available.

The hyperreactivity to mold toxins in these patients tends to be very high, requiring extreme measures in order for them to get clear enough to make much progress toward recovery.

Less severely ill patients are usually less reactive and thus may require less extreme measures in order to get clear of exposure levels harmful to them.

Nonetheless, we suggest that following the basic principles outlined in this book may result in the maximum and most long-lasting improvements for them as well.

Going Forward

As treatment options go, mold avoidance is a particularly challenging path to follow.

Only because it has been effective in facilitating improvements when nothing else has worked has anyone been willing to pursue it.

It is our hope that as a result of our sharing information about this approach more widely in this book, researchers and clinicians will become interested in the mold hyperreactivity phenomenon as well as in the toxicity component of the illness.

Perhaps if this occurs, other treatments for existing patients as well as effective prevention strategies will emerge.

About the Photos

The photos in this book were taken by Lisa during her travels seeking out good locations in the western half of the US from 2009-2014.

Although there is no guarantee that all of these locations will be good ones now or into the future, they all felt excellent to her when the photos were taken.

Disclaimer

The information in this book is based on our own experiences and on the anecdotal reports of hundreds of other mold avoiders who have shared their experiences with us.

Because "science" has yet to demonstrate any interest in the mold hyperreactivity phenomenon, we cannot provide any guarantees about the extent to which the techniques here will be helpful to others with this kind of disease or about whether our comments will turn out to be representative of the underlying truth of the illness.

We are making the information available only so that others who might find it interesting or helpful will have access to it, as well as with the hope that our sharing it will lead to more systematic research into its validity.

Lisa Petrison
Erik Johnson
May 2015

Part 1

BASICS

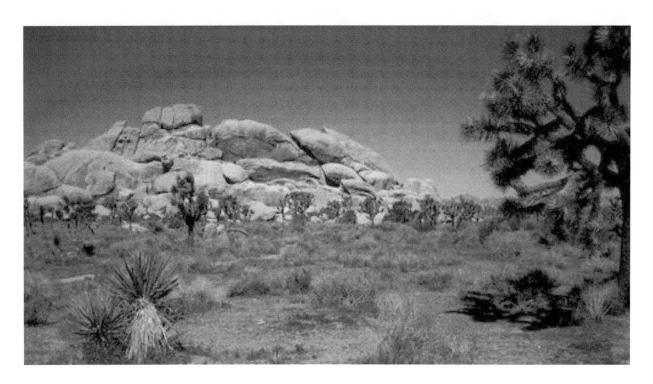

Joshua Tree National Park in the California desert.

Chapter 1

Background

Here is some background information about topics related to mold, mold toxins and mold hyperreactivity.

Mold

Mold is a type of fungus. Its main purpose is to break down substances in the environment.

It is an inherent, natural and necessary part of the world.

The vast majority of mold is not toxic.

Although non-toxic mold can trigger allergic reactions and respiratory problems, it is not the focus of the health issues discussed in this book.

Mold Toxins

A very few species of mold produce certain chemicals that are harmful to humans and to other animals.

These chemicals are called mycotoxins.

Mycotoxins are not alive. They fall into the same category as spider venom.

They are poisons made by living things.

Mycotoxins can be made by toxic molds growing in a wide variety of places -- for instance, in the outdoors, in buildings, in sewers, in foods, and (possibly) in the human body.

There are many thousands of papers in the peer-reviewed literature detailing the negative health effects of exposure to these chemicals.

Aflatoxin is an accepted cause of liver cancer.

Ochratoxin is known to damage kidneys.

Penitrem A has been shown to cause channelopathies leading to neurological damage and heart problems.

Trichothecenes are acknowledged to cause harm to the immune system, the neurological system and the intestinal tract.

Other Substances

In addition to mycotoxins, mold is known to be able to produce a few other potentially dangerous substances.

The volatile organic compounds (VOC's) made by mold are different than the mycotoxins but have been shown to have the ability to cause neurological damage.

Molds are recognized as having the ability to transform metals into their nanoparticle forms.

The proteins in mold spores can trigger negative reactions as well.

The extent to which all of these substances may be involved in chronic multisystem illness has yet to be studied and remains unclear.

Mold Hyperreactivity

Mycotoxins have the potential to cause harm to anyone if exposure is great enough.

It is believed by some mold specialists that most people have genetics that provide them with some protection against suffering long-run damage from mycotoxins, even if they get substantial exposure.

Most of the rest of the population can get some limited exposure to mycotoxins without experiencing substantial harm.

Unfortunately, a small percentage of people appear unable to get new exposures to even very small amounts of certain mold toxins without experiencing substantial harm as a result.

Anecdotally, it seems that many of these individuals previously have endured extended exposures to environments that were particularly problematic with regard to toxic mold.

When these hyperreactive individuals are exposed to even small amounts of these toxins on an ongoing basis, their illness symptoms present in ways that are appropriately diagnosed as myalgic encephalomyelitis, chronic Lyme disease, Gulf War illness, fibromyalgia or other related diseases.

When these people decrease their exposures to these toxins to a level that does not cause them harm, their symptoms begin to recede.

Decreased exposures to these toxins also may allow their bodies to be more able to engage in activities such as detoxification, pathogen killing and systems repair.

The goal of mold avoidance is to decrease exposures to mold toxins to levels low enough that health symptoms decrease and healing starts to occur.

Does This Mean Avoiding All Mold?

For most people who have become hyperreactive to mold toxins, avoiding all mold is not desirable or necessary.

The goal is to avoid only those toxins that are prompting a hyperreactivity reaction.

A minority of people who become hyperreactive to mold toxins also have reported experiencing an anaphylactic-type reaction to what may be the protein in mold spores (including the spores of non-toxic mold), similar to the way that some people become reactive to peanuts or latex.

This may require avoidance of all mold and is a more difficult undertaking.

Other Microbial Toxins

Mold is not the only type of microorganism that can make toxins damaging to humans.

Certain bacteria growing in water-damaged buildings may produce toxins with similar effects to those made by toxic molds.

Certain species of aquatic microorganisms such as cyanobacteria and diatoms have been found to make very damaging toxins as well.

Individuals who are hyperreactive to mold toxins tend to be hyperreactive to other kinds of microbial toxins as well.

The toxins made by these varied microorganisms may be synergistic in their effects, meaning that combinations of toxins may be much more damaging than single toxins.

Causality

Although hyperreactivity to toxins made by mold and other microbes has been reported by many hundreds of patients, it has yet to receive any published scientific study.

Thus, the percentage of patients with myalgic encephalomyelitis, chronic Lyme disease, Gulf War illness, fibromyalgia or similar illnesses who are hyperreactive to toxic mold has yet to be determined.

Anecdotally, nearly all of those individuals with these diagnoses who have tried mold avoidance according to the precepts in this book have concluded that mold hyperreactivity is an issue for them and that they are better off pursuing mold avoidance insofar as they are reasonably able to do so.

Whether this observation would hold with a larger sample remains to be seen.

Even if every single sufferer of these diseases were found to be hyperreactive to toxic mold, that would not necessarily implicate toxic mold as a cause of any of the diseases.

It could be that something else is causal, with the reactivities to toxic mold purely downstream.

Many people do report first becoming hyperreactive to mold toxins while living or working in an environment that is particularly contaminated with toxic mold.

However, without formal study, it is impossible to know whether exposure to toxic mold is a risk factor for becoming hyperreactive to it or for getting any of these diseases.

Even if toxic mold makes it more likely that individuals will get sick with one of these illnesses, additional factors (such as genetic predisposition, the presence of one or more specific pathogens in the system, exposures to other environmental agents, physical injury or a specific nutritional deficiency) probably are needed in order to make mold-related illness manifest in a specific way.

Pursuing Avoidance

Regardless of whether toxic mold is a cause of their health symptoms, individuals who are hyperreactive to mold toxins may benefit from decreasing their exposure to those toxins.

People do not have to believe that gluten or other trigger foods are a cause of their myalgic encephalomyelitis, chronic Lyme disease, Gulf War illness or fibromyalgia in order to benefit from eliminating those foods from their diets.

Similarly, if toxic mold exposures are serving as a trigger that make people feel worse, then eliminating those exposures may help them to feel better.

Disclaimer & Safety Issues

Those considering pursuing mold avoidance of any sort need to be sure to read the disclaimer and safety issues discussion in this book.

It is located at the very end of the book, so that it can be easily found.

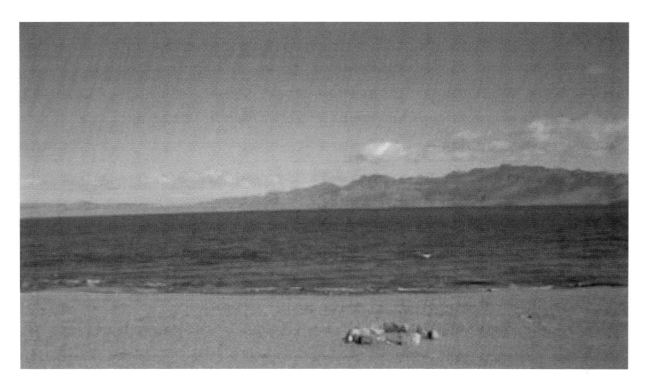

Pyramid Lake near Reno, Nevada.

Chapter 2

History

The use of mold avoidance to address chronic multisystem illness as described in this book was first developed by Erik Johnson.

Erik is a survivor of the 1980's Lake Tahoe epidemic of the very severe illness (appropriately diagnosed as myalgic encephalomyelitis) that eventually was misleadingly named "chronic fatigue syndrome" by the CDC.

During the 1970's, while serving as a nuclear missile launcher specialist in the US Army, Erik received intensive training in how to deal with exposures to dangerous substances (such as nuclear radiation or nerve gas).

Erik was taught that extended exposures to even tiny amounts of these substances (such as the amount that stuck to hair or clothing) could create severe symptoms.

Paying close attention to one's own reactions in order to detect exposures -- and then using avoidance and decontamination techniques to become clear of those exposures -- is the best way to survive in conditions of hazardous environmental toxicity of a variety of different types, the military officers stated.

Although Erik was aware during the 1980's that environmental molds were having a negative effect on him, he experienced only a partial recovery by avoiding them in what seemed to be "reasonable" ways.

In the late 1990's, Erik decided to use the approach that he had learned while serving in the Army to try to get clear of even tiny amounts of certain indoor and outdoor substances that he believed were being made by molds and having a very negative effect on him.

As a result, he experienced a functional recovery (including the ability to work full-time and exercise vigorously), which he has maintained since that time.

Erik subsequently taught a number of other very ill people how to practice his approach effectively, and a few of these have gone on to teach it to others.

Eventually certain mold physicians began recommending a very simplified version of Erik's approach to their patients as well.

Hundreds of individuals with chronic multisystem illness now have benefited by using these mold avoidance techniques.

Erik Johnson's Story

A full history of Erik life is presented in the book *Back from the Edge*, written by Lisa Petrison.

It is available on the Amazon.com website.

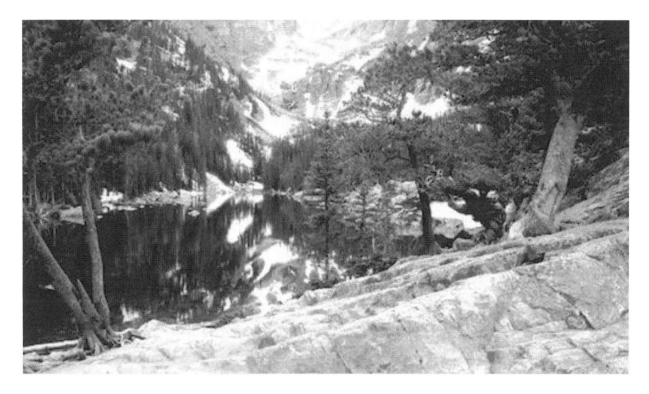

Dream Lake in Rocky Mountain National Park in Colorado.

Chapter 3

Overview

The goal of mold avoidance is to allow those who are hyperreactive to mold toxins to become free of exposures to problematic amounts of those toxins.

This will give their systems a chance to calm down, rather than to continue to experience the constant negative effects of inflammation and other toxin-related harm.

The individual's own personal reactions to the toxins are used a guide for whether exposure is occurring.

This means that it is important to get as free of these toxins as possible at the beginning of the mold avoidance process, so that it will be possible to know when exposures are taking place.

These efforts to become especially free of exposures to mold toxin are referred to in this book as the mold avoidance sabbatical.

Once the system has a chance to get clear of problematic toxins for an extended period of time (preferably for at least a couple of weeks) on the sabbatical, re-exposures tend to have much more immediately noticeable effects.

Those observed effects can be used to determine when exposures are occurring, so that more effective avoidance can take place.

This approach allows those pursuing mold avoidance to avoid only those places or objects that actually are problems for them, rather than to have to guess whether particular places or objects conceivably might be a problem.

Those pursuing mold avoidance in this way thus can lead much more normal lives than they would if they were avoiding all suspect places or objects "just in case."

Using this approach also facilitates more effective avoidance, since it is rarely the case that anyone can predict with any great degree of accuracy whether a particular location, building or object is likely to be free of problematic mold toxins.

In order to accomplish the goal of decreasing toxic exposures to a low enough level not to trigger the hyperreactivity response, specific tactics have been found to be helpful.

One important tactic involves establishing a safe space that is as free of toxins as possible and then protecting it against cross-contaminations.

Many mold avoiders use decontamination techniques (such as showering and changing clothes) to protect themselves from extended effects of toxins subsequent to being exposed to them.

Making an effort to become very clear of toxins during discrete periods of time may allow larger amounts of toxins to be endured without negative effects at other times.

These and other approaches to managing the hyperreactivity component of the illness and moving toward healing are discussed in the remainder of this book.

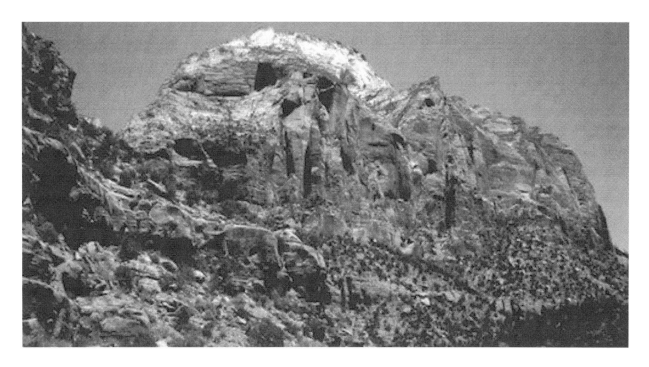

Zion National Park in southern Utah.

Chapter 4

Hyperreactivity

The hyperreactivity phenomenon is at the basis of pursuing mold avoidance.

Some people are affected particularly strongly when they encounter even tiny amounts of the toxins made by certain molds.

If people are very hyperreactive and the toxins are very problematic, then even incredibly small amounts of exposure can be enough to keep them wholly sick.

By staying clear of even those tiny amounts of toxins, people can avoid being negatively affected by them and thus make health gains.

Severity of Reactions

Likely the biggest challenge in practicing mold avoidance successfully is accepting the concept that for some people, even ridiculously tiny exposures can produce unreasonably large effects.

For instance, it seems reasonable to think that someone who is hyperreactive to toxic mold might not do well eating lunch in a moldy restaurant.

What seems more unreasonable is the idea that after spending 30 seconds in that moldy restaurant, the person might become more and more sick for hours after leaving -- just from the cross-contamination on hair and clothing.

It seems reasonable to think that people might be harmed by living in a moldy home.

What seems more unreasonable is to think that chairs in a doctor's office might be so cross-contaminated by patients living in moldy homes that they cannot be used by hyperreactive individuals without triggering symptoms.

It seems reasonable to think that some factories in Asia might be toxic enough to be causing illness in their workers.

What seems more unreasonable is to think that a computer made in one of those factories might be cross-contaminated enough with problematic toxins to trigger severe illness all by itself.

It seems reasonable to accept that living in a city with toxic air might have health dangers.

What seems more unreasonable is to accept that a car that spent a month in a city with toxic air years ago might have become toxic enough from that exposure to cause symptoms in people standing 20 yards away from the vehicle.

And yet, the level of reactivity described in these "unreasonable" examples is reported regularly by patients who were previously very ill and who have improved substantially since starting mold avoidance.

Hyperreactivity that is this extreme makes mold avoidance a challenge.

Nevertheless, many people with this level of hyperreactivity have successfully pursued mold avoidance to the point where they have benefited substantially.

Some of them also have eventually reduced their reactivity so that they no longer have to be as scrupulous in their avoidance activities.

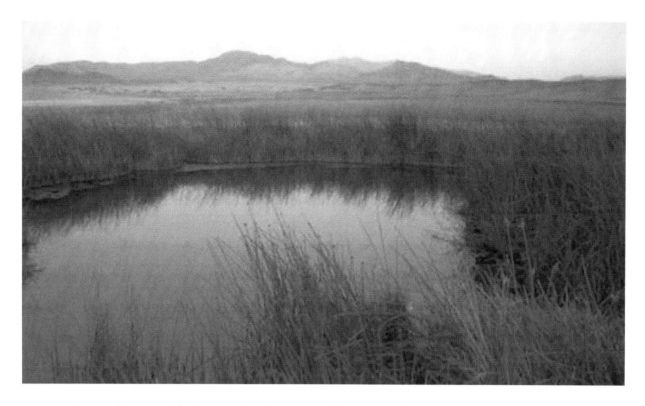

An outdoor mud bath near the tiny town of Tecopa in the eastern California desert.

Chapter 5

Skeptics

The idea that people can be so hyperreactive to toxic mold that even the tiniest exposure can drop them in their tracks is very hard for most people to believe.

The skepticism does not seem to be due to doubts about the idea that tiny amounts of certain substances can cause severe reactions. There are many substances -- such as latex, peanuts and gluten -- that are firmly acknowledged to do so.

The idea that mycotoxins are capable of causing health harm is not that hard to believe either.

There are thousands of papers on that in the medical literature.

The main issue that seems to prompt skepticism is the idea that - since the world is filled with molds of various sorts - a person who is unable to tolerate mold would seem unable to live in the world at all.

Skeptics ask, "Wouldn't that be what life would be like for someone with a severe peanut allergy, if the world were covered in peanut dust? How could that person survive?"

Part of the answer to this question lies in the fact that most mold does not make toxins.

In addition, not all mold toxins are equally bad.

Avoiding just the mold toxins that are problematic enough to cause major negative effects in extremely tiny amounts is much easier than avoiding all mold or all mold toxins.

However, it is true that a relatively high percentage of buildings, locations and objects are affected by mold toxins that are problematic enough to have a negative effect on hyperreactive individuals even in fairly small amounts.

That's why mold avoidance is so difficult.

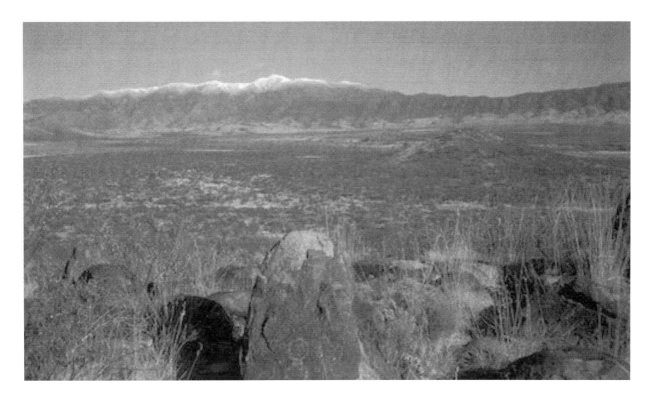

City of Rocks State Park near Silver City, New Mexico.

Chapter 6

Masking

People who are very hyperreactive to toxic mold almost invariably have no idea that it is affecting them at all.

This is largely due to the fact that if the body is exposed to a problematic substance on a continual basis, it will stop reacting acutely and instead do its best to cope with the exposure.

This is called masking.

The phenomenon of masking is well-accepted with regard to gluten sensitivities or other food intolerances.

If someone is suspicious about whether they might be reacting to gluten, then the generally accepted best way to find out for sure whether it is an issue is to remove all traces of it from the diet for a few weeks.

If gluten indeed is a problem, the negative effects of it will be much more noticeable when it is reintroduced into the diet after a vacation from it.

Living in a moldy house, day in and day out, is the same principle as eating gluten at every meal.

Without any break from the problem substance, the body will deal with it as well as it can.

Especially for someone living in a bad environment, it takes effort to avoid toxic mold to the degree necessary to get clear.

But until people get clear, they have no way of knowing whether they are reacting to toxic mold at all.

All that they generally know is that they are sick, for no apparent reason.

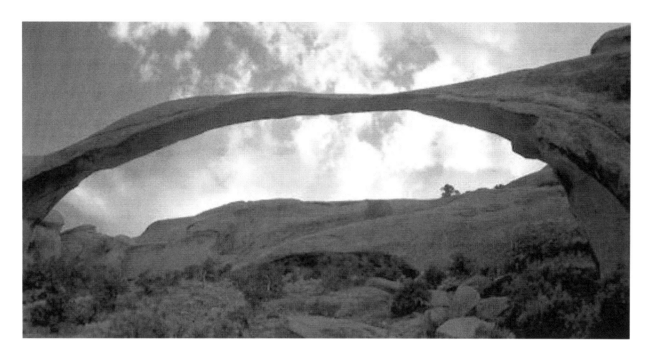

Landscape Arch at Arches National Park near Moab, Utah.

Chapter 7

Sources of Exposure

In order to get clear of mold toxins to the extent needed to effectively practice mold avoidance, several different sources of exposure need to be consistently considered.

These include building toxins, outdoor toxins, cross-contaminated possessions, and personal cross-contamination.

Tap water is not infrequently contaminated with biotoxins and can cause problems as well.

Any of these exposure types has the potential of keeping people who are hyperreactive to mold toxins wholly ill.

Moving into even the most mold-free house on the planet may not make one bit of noticeable difference if the outdoor air is a problem or if cross-contamination makes its way into the environment.

Some hyperreactive individuals do luck into environments that are good enough for them, without specifically thinking about (say) outdoor air.

Insofar as the goal is to maximize the likelihood of seeing improvements via mold avoidance though, keeping all of these possible sources of exposure in mind may be beneficial.

Building Mold

Toxic mold that grows in buildings is an increasingly recognized health threat.

The prevalence of toxic molds growing indoors has skyrocketed since building styles changed in the late 1970's (to include such factors as drywall, increased insulation, decreased air circulation and HVAC systems).

The subsequent explosion of cases of diseases such as myalgic encephalomyelitis, fibromyalgia and chronic Lyme may be at least in part a result of the mold growth resulting from these changes in building styles.

Toxic mold in buildings often grows inside drywall or in wall insulation, where it often cannot be seen or smelled.

Trichothecenes also have been shown to disrupt the ability of the brain to detect odors, making it less likely that individuals will have the ability to smell mold even when it is growing in the open.

Therefore, people who are being exposed to severe toxic mold problems frequently are totally unaware that there is any problem with mold in the building at all.

Even when Stachybotrys (a mold with strong neurological and immunological effects) can be seen, it tends to look more like smears of dirt on the wall than what most people would think of as mold.

Another problem is that most conventional mold tests are highly inaccurate, especially when it comes to identifying the presence of Stachybotrys.

The ERMI and HERTSMI-2 tests are more reliable but have been reported by some individuals to have missed serious mold growth problems as well.

Outdoor Mold

Outdoor environments typically include a wide variety of different types of mold, most of them non-toxic.

However, many mold avoiders have found that there are some outdoor toxins that have the ability to keep them just as sick as they would be if they were living in a very bad building.

Some of the outdoor toxins that are most problematic for those hyperreactive to mold toxins seem to be especially associated with sewage (such as city sewers or sewer ponds) or composting facilities.

Fire retardants, certain agricultural chemicals (especially glyphosate) and industrial solvent spills also seem to be associated with the presence of outdoor toxins problematic for those individuals who are hyperreactive to mold toxins.

For the most part, the chemicals themselves do not seem to be the major issue.

Problems more seem to occur when microorganisms are growing in close proximity to the chemicals.

Certain algae growing in oceans, lakes, rivers and ponds also have the ability to make airborne biotoxins that can be problematic for people who are hyperreactive to mold toxins.

All of these outdoor toxins have the potential of blowing long distances, meaning that they can be problematic for hyperreactive individuals far from the source points.

These toxins usually make their way into indoor environments in affected locations and in many cases cannot be effectively filtered from the indoor air with available technologies.

Cross-Contaminated Objects

Many people tend to have an inherent belief that simply moving out of a particularly problematic environment will result in at least some health gains.

Very frequently, that is not what happens for individuals with moderate or severe chronic multisystem illness.

Insofar as hyperreactive individuals bring their possessions from a bad environment with them to their new environment, the cross-contamination on those items has the potential of keeping them just as ill as they were when still living in the problematic place.

Even transitory exposure to a bad environment or to other cross-contaminated objects sometimes can be enough to cause a particular object to become contaminated enough to keep a hyperreactive individual totally sick.

While washing items sometimes may be helpful, in many cases this does not resolve the problem for those individuals who are hyperreactive to mold toxins.

Many people have found that discarding all their possessions or putting them in long-term storage has been necessary for them to be able to recover any substantial amount of their health after moving from a particularly problematic environment.

The longer that items have been exposed to environments with particularly problematic toxic mold growth, the more difficult those items tend to be to remediate.

Casual contaminations tend to be more likely to be able to be washed off successfully.

Personal Cross-Contamination

When people visit problematic buildings or locations, the toxin-laden spores or spore fragments stick to their hair, clothing and skin.

This level of exposure can be enough to keep hyperreactive people very ill for many hours or days.

Removing these toxins by showering and changing to uncontaminated clothing can be helpful in stopping the reactions.

Water

Some locations obtain their water supply from lakes or rivers contaminated with cyanobacteria toxins.

These toxins are rarely filtered out by water departments and therefore may be present in tap water.

Hyperreactive people may be negatively affected by these toxins, not just from drinking the water but also from using it to shower or to wash objects.

Considering how to obtain reliably uncontaminated water for both drinking and washing purposes may be worthwhile.

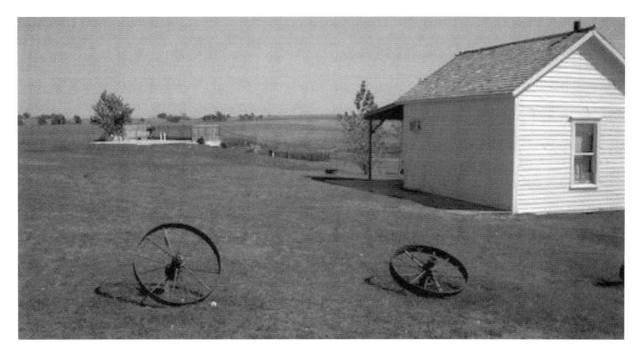

The Laura Ingalls Wilder family farm, just outside De Smet, South Dakota.

Chapter 8

Toxins

People with mold hyperreactivity react negatively to a variety of different toxins.

Some of these toxins have much worse effects than others on these individuals.

Most of those mold avoiders who have been the most successful in reclaiming a reasonable life have adopted a strategy whereby they are particularly scrupulous with regard to avoiding those toxic substances that have very bad effects on them.

These successful mold avoiders usually also try to make an effort to avoid toxic substances that have milder effects on them, but not necessarily quite so scrupulously.

Super Toxins

It frequently has been reported that here are some toxins that have the ability to keep hyperreactive individuals totally sick, even in very tiny quantities.

Cross-contamination of a single object in a home with one of these toxins would be sufficient keep some hyperreactive people from recovering at all, for example.

These particularly problematic toxins appear to be consistent in triggering very negative effects in all people hyperreactive to toxic mold, rather than in just a subset of those individuals.

Anecdotal observations suggest that people with chronic multisystem diseases (such as myalgic encephalomyelitis, chronic Lyme disease, fibromyalgia or multiple chemical sensitivities) very often become ill in buildings containing substantial amounts of these super toxins.

Often these individuals continue to be exposed to unusually high levels of these super toxins on a continual basis for many years after getting sick.

Even if they move away from the problematic building or location, the cross-contamination on possessions can provide an ongoing source of exposure.

Anecdotally, these super toxins appear to usually originate from sewers or from buildings.

Only occasionally do they seem to originate from other outdoor areas.

Super toxins seem especially likely to emerge in circumstances where microbial growth (such as mold) is present in places where certain toxic chemicals (such as industrial solvents, fire retardants, adhesives or flea bombs) have been used.

In some cases, super toxins appear to be associated with recognized toxic molds such as Stachybotrys.

However, while Stachybotrys is known to be present in at least small amounts in a high percentage of buildings, super toxins are much more uncommon.

This suggests the possibility that Stachybotrys only manufactures the super toxin a certain percentage of the time, or that another microbe that sometimes grows in conjunction with Stachybotrys is responsible for making the super toxin.

None of the published literature on the health effects of specific mycotoxins appears to have looked at super toxins.

The literature looks instead at toxins that are commonly made by toxic molds and that do not have the magnified effects of the super toxins.

Commercially available environmental mold tests (including the ERMI) look only at the types of molds present in an environment rather than at the particular toxins being made by those molds.

They therefore present no solid information about the extent to which any particular toxins are present or absent.

Because super toxins have been observed to be relatively unusual and to have a very deleterious effect on hyperreactive individuals even in tiny quantities, focusing particular attention on avoiding them scrupulously may be worthwhile.

Observations suggest that a high percentage of individuals with chronic multisystem illness are being exposed to problematic amounts of super toxins on a continual basis (from their home, their location or their belongings).

These individuals almost invariably believe that toxic exposures have nothing to do with their illness and that their problems come from "within."

Only after they get clear of their usual environments and possessions for a period of time do these individuals realize what a negative effect these very powerful toxins have been having on them.

Regular Toxic Mold

Regular toxic molds are accepted by science as being present in almost all buildings, in many outdoor environments, and in many foods.

The toxins made by these molds have been studied extensively, with many thousands of peer-reviewed papers showing negative health effects resulting from exposures to them.

The effects have been especially studied in the agricultural literature, looking at the effects on animals of mycotoxins ingested through contaminated feed.

Early skepticism about the ability of mycotoxins in buildings to cause similar health effects rested on the assumption that the total amount of mycotoxins taken into the system would be much larger from eating moldy food than breathing moldy air.

The injuries that people get from living or working in moldy buildings now tend to be explained as being related to the following research findings.

a) Toxins are generally much more dangerous when inhaled than when ingested.

b) Combinations of toxins (e.g. mold, bacterial, chemical) in sick buildings often are synergistic in their effects.

c) The effects of satratoxin trichothecenes (made by Stachybotrys) are substantially stronger than the effects of the Fusarium trichothecenes that are commonly present in animal feed.

An additional possibility is that the really problematic super toxins that have been observed to be associated with environments where people get sick with mold illness have not yet been studied in the literature.

Perhaps it is these super toxins (rather than the regular mold toxins that have been studied at length) that are responsible for people falling ill with chronic multisystem illness in certain buildings.

Hopefully this possibility eventually will be examined in a systematic way.

Regardless of whether regular mold toxins in buildings have the ability in themselves to cause healthy people to fall ill with chronic multisystem illness, they certainly have the potential to have very negative effects even in fairly small quantities on hyperreactive individuals.

The ERMI test (which looks at household dust to determine via genetic analysis the species of mold that are present) is designed to determine the extent to which various regular toxic molds are growing in buildings.

Although a number of individuals with chronic multisystem illness have reported that the ERMI has not picked up on substantial mold problems in their homes, the test does seem to have the ability to effectively identify most buildings with large amounts of problematic toxic mold growth.

For people who are hyperreactive to mold toxins, avoiding buildings that are particularly problematic with regard to regular toxic molds certainly is a good idea.

Decreasing total exposure to these regular toxic molds to very low levels also has been reported as helpful by many mold avoiders, especially those who are severely hyperreactive.

Still, reports from mold avoiders suggest that even tiny exposures to certain unusual super toxins can be much more detrimental to them than living in a house that has moderate amounts of regular toxic mold.

Non-Toxic Mold

A small percentage of mold avoiders report being reactive to all mold, whether toxic or non-toxic.

In some cases, the reported reaction to non-toxic mold is inflammation similar to that associated with toxic mold.

This type of reaction tends to be especially prevalent early in avoidance when people are very hyperreactive.

Possibly it is related to the presence of mildly toxic poisons present even in mold that is officially considered "non-toxic."

In addition, a small minority of individuals who are hyperreactive to mold toxins develop reactions to what may be the proteins in the mold spores.

These reactions tend to manifest similarly to anaphylactic allergies (such as the kind that some people have to peanuts or latex) or to affect the respiratory tract.

Being very reactive to all mold rather than just to mold toxins can make mold avoidance much more difficult.

Some people with this issue have found that they are able to stay well only in special housing in isolated and very dry areas, for example.

Insofar as reactions to non-toxic molds are being driven by an allergy of some sort, it is possible that allergy or autoimmune treatments might be helpful.

Unfortunately, those kinds of treatments have yet to be reported to us to be helpful with hyperreactivities to mold toxins.

Some reports suggest that they even may be counterproductive for that.

Chemicals

A high percentage of people who are hyperreactive to the chemicals made by toxic molds also are especially reactive to manmade chemicals.

Some of these individuals also report being hyperreactive to mercury or to other heavy metals; to the chemicals made by certain plants (such as terpenes); to smoke of all kinds; and to other natural substances.

Insofar as chemical substances of any sort are prompting problematic reactions, avoiding them to the extent necessary to stop the reactions seems like a good idea.

Anecdotally, mold toxins tend to cross-contaminate much more than manmade chemicals do.

In addition, people are much less likely to spontaneously figure out on their own that they are being exposed to problematic biotoxins than that they are being exposed to other problematic chemicals.

People who find themselves reactive to mold toxins often begin reducing the amount of other chemicals in their environments, either because of their reactivities to those chemicals or because it seems like a generally good idea.

Many mold avoiders have reported that their reactivities to chemicals have dropped substantially after many months or years of scrupulous mold avoidance.

In many cases chemical reactivities have increased for a period of time early in mold avoidance, however.

For those who are severely sensitive to chemicals other than those made by mold, a variety of resources on the topics of environmental illness (EI) or multiple chemical sensitivity (MCS) are available.

However, even when these resources bring up the topic of environmental mold, their instructions on how to handle it should not be anticipated to provide much help to those who have become especially hyperreactive to mold toxins.

According to the reports of many mold avoiders, individuals who are engaging in extreme measures to avoid chemical triggers very frequently are living unknowingly with constant exposures to particularly problematic super toxins.

These exposures may include contamination of belongings with super toxins, living in places with very problematic outdoor air, or residing in particularly bad buildings or RV's.

Many of those mold avoiders who have looked into "MCS-safe housing" offered by individuals who define themselves as having environmental illness have found a high percentage of those housing alternatives to be affected substantially by the worst kinds of mold toxins.

Individuals with MCS often may provide information inappropriate to mold avoiders about whether particular locations are good as well.

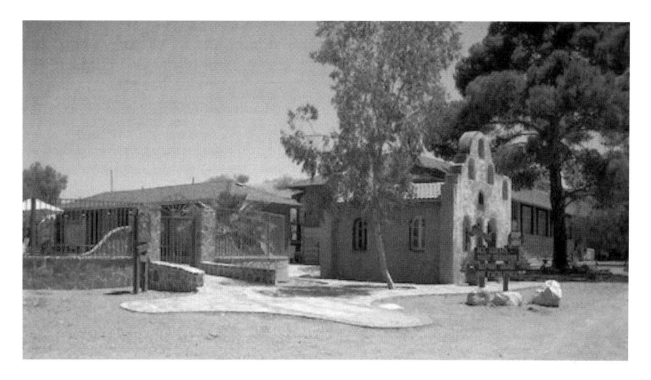

Mercey Hot Springs, near Los Banos, California.

Chapter 9

Unmasking

Unmasking from toxic mold involves the same basic concept as unmasking from gluten or other suspected dietary triggers.

The first step is to spend an extended period of time getting as free as possible from the substance in question.

Some people have found that a week has been sufficient to get them unmasked enough to start out, though this is generally not ideal.

Spending two weeks or more on this sort of sabbatical is better.

Even if a hyperreactive individual actually gets clear of the problematic substance during the avoidance sabbatical, that person may not feel better during that time.

A few people have reported feeling dramatically better within just a few days of getting clear.

Many others have reported that they did not feel much different during the sabbatical.

Some people have reported that in some respects (especially with regard to heavy fatigue, chemical sensitivities or fibromyalgia-type pain), they actually felt worse while on the sabbatical than in what they eventually realized was a very toxic home environment.

Regardless of how people feel during the mold avoidance sabbatical, the real benefit of going through it comes upon the return to the usual environment.

This is similar to how the real test of whether people are sensitive to gluten occurs when the person reintroduces wheat back into the diet and then observes whether there is a noticeable negative effect.

Provided that people actually get clear of problematic toxins during the sabbatical, they should be able to tell whether they are reacting to those toxins when they come back into contact with them after the sabbatical is over.

They then can use those reactions to effectively avoid problematic toxins in the future.

Insofar as these individuals continue to avoid problematic substances to the extent that their hyperreactivity requires, substantial health improvements generally begin to become apparent within anywhere from a few days to a few months.

Part 2

AVOIDANCE SABBATICAL

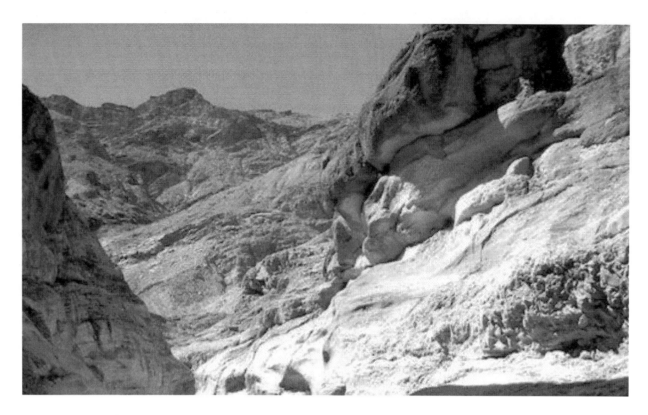

Hiking Mosaic Canyon in Death Valley National Park in eastern California.

Chapter 10

The Sabbatical

Observations suggest that a very high percentage of people with chronic multisystem illness are living in situations where they are getting substantial exposure to unusually problematic super toxins.

Observations also suggest that insofar as hyperreactive individuals are being exposed to these super toxins, they may have a difficult time making much sustainable health progress regardless of what else they do.

A main goal of the mold avoidance sabbatical is to ensure that individuals get as free as possible of all exposures to these super toxins.

If this is not accomplished, then the whole experiment likely will end up being a waste of time and expenditures.

All sources of these super toxins (including buildings, outside air, possessions and personal cross-contamination) need to be addressed if the experiment is to be a success.

In addition, getting as clear as possible of regular mold toxins during the sabbatical is a worthwhile goal.

While staying in a non-pristine building containing a moderate amount of regular toxic mold may not totally negate the value of the experiment, the results will be clearer if exposures to all kinds of mold toxins are as low as possible.

The mold toxins and other pollution present in the outdoor air in most cities and many agricultural areas constitute a less-than-ideal environment for a mold avoidance sabbatical as well.

Planning the Sabbatical

New mold avoiders have had successful sabbaticals in a variety of different living environments.

These have included homes or hotels judged to be good by individuals already practicing mold avoidance; KOA cabins; converted cargo trailers; and tents.

At least as important as choosing the right lodging is making sure that cross-contamination from the home environment is properly eliminated.

Ensuring that the location chosen for the sabbatical is not particularly toxic also is very important.

Finally, using effective decontamination techniques during the sabbatical can make a big difference in terms of its usefulness.

After the Sabbatical

After a successful sabbatical, hyperreactive individuals become more able to judge whether environments or objects are safe for them, based solely on their own immediate reactions.

They then can focus their avoidance efforts on those toxins that their bodies are alerting them are particularly problematic for them personally.

In most cases, people who have been chronically exposed to super toxins will respond strongly to those toxins after a sabbatical from them, even if they do not get totally clear of all mold toxins during the sabbatical.

As people continue to avoid all substances that trigger their reactions, the ability to identify additional toxins that are somewhat less problematic for them tends to emerge.

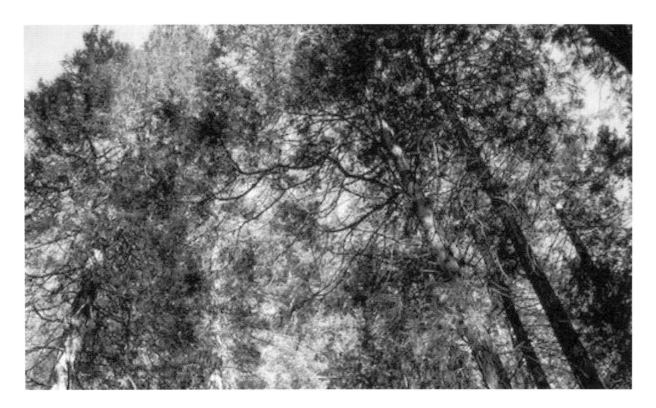

Near California Hot Springs, California.

Chapter 11

Intensification Response

Subsequent to a successful mold avoidance sabbatical, acute reactions to toxins tend to feel much worse than they did prior to getting away.

For the most part, having this happen is the desired outcome of the sabbatical.

Insofar as people experience noticeable reactions to toxins, avoiding those toxins scrupulously becomes much easier.

Unfortunately, especially for people with severe chronic multisystem illness, reactions sometimes can become scarily intense.

The most frequently reported re-exposure symptom has been severe suicidal inclination.

Other particularly problematic symptoms have included passing out, temporary paralysis, inability to speak, seizures or convulsions.

Reports suggest that getting away from the exposure usually allows these symptoms to recede fairly quickly.

In addition, patients who experience these particularly severe symptoms almost always have experienced similar ones in their illness prior to trying avoidance.

However, the potential for reactions to toxins to get worse after an avoidance sabbatical makes it essential for people to consider carefully in advance what they will do if their current residence (or their current possessions or their entire current location) should feel intolerable to them upon their return.

Especially for severely ill individuals, it might be extremely difficult to find a home that does not feel intolerable subsequent to an avoidance sabbatical.

While some people are lucky enough to find conventional housing in that they can tolerate and live in while moving toward recovery, others spend many months or even years searching for a place that feels tolerable to them.

Reported Experiences

The extent to which hyperreactive people experience intensification reaction subsequent to an avoidance sabbatical varies across individuals.

Those with classic ME symptoms (especially very severe fatigue and severe exercise intolerance) often experience particularly dramatic responses when re-exposed.

Other mold avoiders have stated that they are not convinced that the toxins affected them more negatively after getting clear of them than they did before.

When it occurs, intensification reaction tends to be particularly strong during the first months of avoidance.

Typically, as time goes on, mold avoiders become more able to easily identify toxins in their environments and thus to avoid them more scrupulously.

This may make it seem as though their reactivity is increasing.

However, in most cases these same individuals acknowledge that their overall health (in terms of how they feel and what they can do) is improving and that exposures do not take as much out of them as they did at the beginning.

Some people have suggested that while sensitivity (the ability to identify the toxins based on initial reactions) is going up, reactivity (the tendency to be harmed by the toxins when exposed) is going down.

This may mean that progress is being made even though hyperreactivity remains very high.

The extent to which reactivity decreases over time may be dependent on a variety of factors.

Successful detoxification and successful treatment of pathogens have been cited by many patients as being helpful in reducing their reactivity over time.

In some cases, individuals have stated that they feel that they have remained in the intensification reaction stage indefinitely, with their reactivity coming down slowly over time or not coming down at all.

Avoidance Sabbatical Concerns

Some patients express concerns about the possibility of getting "stuck" in intensification response, rather than having the ability to return to the masked state that they experienced prior to experimenting with avoidance.

Anecdotally, many mold avoiders have spent significant amounts of time in good environments, then moved back to somewhat less good environments.

Those individuals report that after a period of discomfort, their systems seemed to settle back down into objecting less but also with decreased functionality, similar to how they were before getting clear.

We have almost no reports of individuals going on mold avoidance sabbatical and then allowing themselves to be re-exposed to toxins that felt particularly bad to them for extended periods of time.

In virtually all cases, people being exposed to very problematic toxins subsequent to getting clear have been motivated to spend a phenomenal amount of energy to get away from those exposures within a fairly short period of time.

However, many mold avoiders state that they have chosen to allow themselves to be exposed to toxins that were moderately bad for them in order to accomplish other goals (such as being close to family, pursuing a career, having fun or feeling less stressed).

We have encountered virtually no individuals who have successfully gotten clear of toxic mold and found that they were hyperreactive who have stated that they were sorry to have experimented with mold avoidance and wished that they could go back to not knowing whether toxic mold was a factor in their illness.

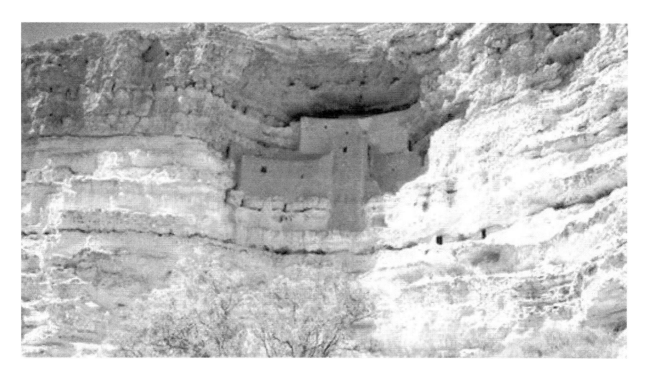

A cliff dwelling at the Montezuma Castle National Monument in northern Arizona.

Chapter 12

Sabbatical Location

Getting as clear as possible for the mold avoidance sabbatical requires careful consideration of three sources of exposure: housing, possessions and location.

Having a decontamination strategy in place to deal with unexpected personal exposures is important as well.

Almost everyone starts out with mold avoidance by underestimating the effects that their location might be having on them.

Only by spending time in a variety of locations do people start to realize what an important factor the locations effect can be for them.

In addition, individuals only will realize that location makes a difference if they are not being exposed to super toxins that have such a negative effect that the positive effects of the good environment are cancelled out.

Those who bring super toxins with them from their problematic usual environment on the sabbatical may not experience any benefits at all.

Depending on people's level of reactivity, some locations are problematic enough with regard to super toxins that they may be wholly inappropriate for an avoidance sabbatical.

Objects such as cars or clothing that have spent time in those particularly problematic locations may best be considered unsuitable as well.

Other locations are less problematic in terms of super toxins but nonetheless have substantial amounts of more ordinary toxins of various sorts (including mold toxins).

Most cities fall into this category, as would many agricultural areas.

If possible, it would be preferable to choose a particularly good area than a somewhat problematic one for the mold avoidance sabbatical.

However, insofar as a particularly good area is not a viable option, an average or even below-average location in terms of regular mold toxins and other pollution may be sufficient to allow people to get clear enough from super toxins to be able to identify those super toxins based on their own reactions to them when re-exposed.

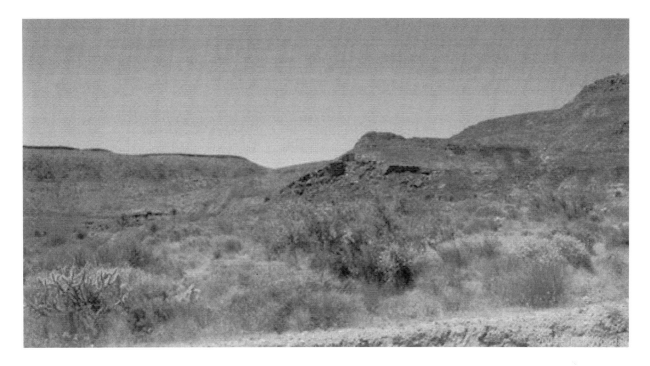

The Mojave National Preserve in the California desert.

Chapter 13

Sabbatical Possessions

Unfortunately, some toxins are so problematic for severe reactors that even one contaminated object in a living space can be enough to keep those individuals totally sick.

A main goal in doing a sabbatical is to determine whether any of those particularly bad toxins are present in the individual's usual living environment.

Therefore, a critical component of the avoidance sabbatical test is to get away from the entire usual environment, including possessions.

An added complication is that a high percentage of washing machines (especially public washing machines) are contaminated with a particularly problematic toxin that can ruin the avoidance sabbatical all by itself.

Therefore, consideration of alternative ways of washing clothing, bedding and other fabric items is necessary in order to eliminate this possibility.

Replacement Possessions

A first challenge is figuring out how to obtain possessions to use on the sabbatical.

One consideration is that it may be better not to buy new possessions (especially items such as clothing or bedding) in local stores prior to going on the sabbatical.

If the location of the home environment is suspected of being particularly problematic, then items in stores may be contaminated by toxins in the outdoor air.

In addition, new items have the potential of being inadvertently cross-contaminated by the person planning the avoidance sabbatical as a result of their being handled in the store, transported in the car or stored prior to the trip.

One alternate possibility is to order needed items via mail order and to have them sent to the destination so that they will be available upon arrival.

Choosing a mail order company that has been reliably okay for other experienced mold avoiders may be an additional precaution.

LL Bean has gotten generally good reports, for instance.

Considering the extent to which needed possessions can be purchased at the destination is worth considering as well.

Some people have been successful in pursuing an avoidance sabbatical with borrowed possessions, though this is a bit of a risk.

Preferably these items would be borrowed from someone without symptoms of any diseases that might be related to mold toxicity (e.g. without chronic multisystem illness, autoimmune disorders or psychological illness).

Decontamination

The basic idea is to get to the destination and then to get as clear as possible from any toxins that may have been brought from home.

A basic protocol would be something like the following.

1. Ideally few items would be brought from the home environment. Any items that are brought should be put aside in a place where they will not be encountered during the sabbatical. For instance, this could be in the trunk of the car, outdoors in plastic bins with a tarp over them, or in containers in a garage or closet space. Be aware that if

these items are brought into the planned living space, they may shed toxins that could be a problem even if the contaminated items are then removed.

2. Remove possibly contaminated clothing worn to the sabbatical location and put it in a garbage bag or other plastic bag (to be stored with the other items from home). Again, a goal is to have the planned living space have as little exposure to suspect items as possible. Undressing just inside the front door before heading for the shower -- or taking the initial shower elsewhere -- would be preferable.

3. Take a shower, including washing hair. No special soap or shampoo is required; mild versions actually may be preferable. Especially when some kinds of toxins are a suspected factor, some people suggest rinsing sinuses, soaking in or scrubbing with Epsom salts, or using a brush in the shower.

4. After showering, open the package with the new clothing and put it on. Although new clothing may be contaminated with regular mold toxins, it is much less likely to be contaminated with really problematic toxins than items that individuals with chronic illness have brought from home. Hand washing or rinsing new clothing when possible then can be considered.

Electronics

The most difficult part of the avoidance sabbatical for many people is figuring out what to do about electronics.

The idea of being without access to a computer, the Internet or a telephone for two weeks is hard for most people to accept.

Replacing those items with new ones may be expensive and inconvenient, however.

Some solutions that people have used include the following:

1. Borrow a computer and/or smart phone for the sabbatical from a healthy friend.

2. Use electronics periodically during the trip, outside the living quarters. Designate some of the new clothes to wear only when using the electronics. After each session using the electronics, change and shower before returning to the living space or immediately upon return. Store the clothes worn for using the electronics in a plastic bag between uses if they are not going to be washed immediately.

3. Plan to use publicly available computers (such as may be available in some hotels or copy stores).

4. Depending on the type of toxins suspected to be involved, cleaning an existing smart phone with a wet cloth and putting it into a new case possibly may be deemed acceptable. Staying away from the smart phone except when using it would be a good idea.

Automobile

Insofar as an individual's home environment contains problematic super toxins, then that person's automobile usually will suffer from substantial cross-contamination.

In addition, a few mold avoiders point to a particular car as having been even more problematic than their home environment.

Renting or borrowing a car for the mold sabbatical therefore may be advisable.

If a car is rented or borrowed, storing possibly contaminated possessions in the trunk (preferably in new plastic bins or other containers) would be a good idea, so as not to cross-contaminate the rest of the car.

So would showering and changing into new clothing before getting into the car for the first time.

If it is not possible to obtain a different car for the trial, then the suspect car can be used in a manner similar to the description about electronics.

Certain clothes may be designated for use in the car, with decontamination taking place upon return to the designated safer environment.

Laundry

A particularly bad toxin has been frequently reported as contaminating washing machines.

Dryers associated with contaminated washing machines also tend to be affected.

See Chapter 31 about Hell Toxin for more information on this substance.

Because this toxin is so problematic, making arrangements to hand wash clothing prior to or during the sabbatical is extremely important.

If those arrangements are not made and clothing is instead washed in a contaminated machine, people may not get clear enough during the sabbatical to be able to tell whether mold is an issue for them upon return to the usual environment.

Although new clothing or new linens usually are mildly contaminated before being washed, that contamination is virtually never anywhere near as bad as the contamination that is frequently present in washing machines.

Thus, for the purposes of the sabbatical, it likely would be better not to wash brand new items at all than to wash them in a suspect machine.

Especially during the sabbatical when people are inexperienced, it probably is best to consider the purpose of doing laundry to just rinse off cross-contamination of spores rather than to use special means to remove toxins that may have bonded to the items.

More information about laundry is in Chapter 38.

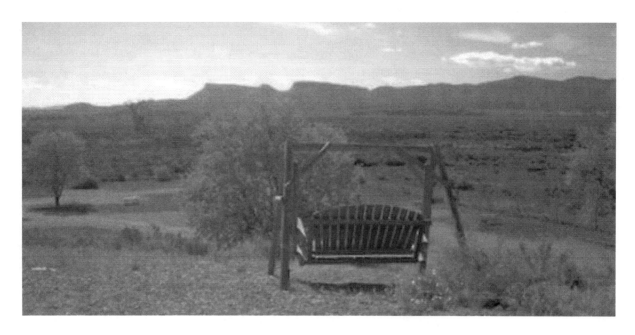

The view from the KOA in Cortez, Colorado.

Chapter 14

Sabbatical Shelter

Finding a shelter that will be good enough with regard to mold toxins for the individual to get relatively clear is the most difficult part about planning the avoidance sabbatical for most people.

Here is a discussion of some different options.

Home of a Friend or Relative

Insofar as a friend or relative has a home that is good enough for a new mold avoider to get relatively clear and is willing to share it for a few weeks, this could be an inexpensive and comfortable option.

The main problem is that it may be very difficult to know for sure whether the home is going to be okay enough for the individual to actually get clear.

Running an environmental mold test such as the ERMI may provide some reassurance with regard to the extent to which toxic mold is growing in the home.

However, that does nothing to ensure that the home is going to be okay in terms of cross-contamination of possessions or the outdoor air.

Therefore, if this option is going to be considered, some guesswork is going to be required.

Perhaps the best clue about the suitability of a particular home is to look at the health of its occupants.

If anyone living in the home has any sort of chronic multisystem disease, then this may not be worth risking for a mold sabbatical.

The exception would be if a chronic multisystem illness patient had experienced substantial improvements in their condition while living in the home.

Buildings where patients with this kind of illness experience substantial recovery very frequently have been found to be quite good.

Health issues such as asthma, other respiratory problems, emotional issues or any kind of "autoimmune" condition experienced by residents of a particular building also may be a clue that an environment may not be good enough to allow hyperreactive individuals to get clear.

Staying with parents may not be a good idea since many mold avoiders have reported their parents' homes to be particularly problematic.

In at least some cases, that could be because exposures to particularly problematic toxins while growing up contributed to the illness manifesting later in life.

Even if parents have moved from a suspect home, their belongings may be cross-contaminated.

Mold avoiders who are struggling with the particularly problematic Hell Toxin (see Chapter 31) often report that the homes of friends or family with whom they have socialized in the past are intolerable for them, due to their having previously cross-contaminated those environments with that super toxin.

Another issue is that often family and friends are located in the same geographic area as the individual.

That means that insofar as outdoor toxins are causing some of the individual's symptoms, there may not be an opportunity to notice a shift.

Nevertheless, it may be the case that staying with friends or family would be so convenient or economical or pleasant that it would be worth considering.

In that case, it may be worthwhile to give it a try - with the understanding that if the sabbatical is not a success, mold hyperreactivity could still be a factor in the illness.

Home of Another Mold Avoider

Insofar as someone with chronic multisystem disease is at a mostly recovered level in a home, then the chances are high that the home is very good with regard to problematic mold toxins.

This is particularly the case if the individual reports still being hyperreactive to other environments.

Whether the home will be tolerable to other individuals in terms of chemical reactivities or non-toxic mold is less certain, since individuals who are hyperreactive to mold toxins may vary in terms of their other reactivities.

Still, in terms of maximizing the likelihood of getting clear of really problematic mold toxins during the sabbatical, this is may be a successful choice.

Unfortunately, this approach has a number of downsides that make it critical that both parties think very carefully about whether it really would be a good idea.

One issue involves cross-contamination.

People who are very ill with chronic multisystem disease and who are not yet practicing avoidance almost invariably are carrying on their person toxins that most people only rarely encounter anywhere else.

Insofar as these toxins are brought into the home of another hyperreactive person, they could have a negative effect on that person's home that could be difficult or impossible for them to remediate to their tolerance level.

In addition, individuals with chronic multisystem illness tend to be susceptible to the same sorts of infections that other sufferers already have.

Insofar as two individuals with this kind of illness are living in the same environment for an extended period of time, the likelihood that they will acquire new infections and thus become more ill may be relatively high.

Another issue is that the mold avoidance sabbatical often is fraught with uncertainty and anxiety.

Especially when individuals are first starting out with avoidance, they may be particularly reactive emotionally.

This can set the stage for a difficult interpersonal situation to occur.

In addition, hosting an ill individual during a sabbatical can require a great deal of time and energy and thus can be a real drain on people who are not wholly well.

If a mostly recovered mold avoider wants to be helpful to someone just starting out, in many cases it might be a better idea for him or her to find a good hotel in the area rather than offering to act as host.

Insofar as new mold avoiders end up doing an avoidance sabbatical at the home of someone already doing avoidance, they may want to consider the idea of paying that individual generously as compensation for the efforts and risks involved.

Hotel

Certain hotels in good locations could be a viable place to do a mold avoidance sabbatical.

The obvious problem is that many hotels have toxic mold problems.

An additional issue is that hotels have many people come through them and thus may be especially likely to be cross-contaminated with particularly problematic toxins.

The likelihood that the washers in hotels will be contaminated with these toxins and that the bedding and towels in the hotel therefore will be especially problematic is high.

However, insofar as individuals can afford to stay in a hotel for an extended period of time and are willing to take the risk that they might not be able to get as clear as they might with other options, a hotel could be worth considering.

Some types of hotels generally are more likely to be better than others.

Hotels with centralized duct systems almost always are problematic, since any toxic issues easily spread throughout the building and since mold may grow inside the ducts.

Hotels with individual window units for heating and cooling for each room tend to be better.

Many mold avoiders have reported that Hampton Inn, Hilton Garden Inn and Doubletree Hotels very often feel good to them, provided that the property was built subsequent to about 2003.

(Hilton flagship hotels may be much more likely to be problematic.)

Asking other mold avoiders for recommendations of hotels that have felt good to them may be a good way to get information on hotels, though obviously some rooms may be better than others or the entire building could go bad.

Bringing sheets and towels to use in the hotel rather than risking the possibility that the ones supplied will be cross-contaminated with particularly problematic toxin is strongly suggested.

KOA Cabins

Kampgrounds of America (KOA) is a commercial campground chain.

In addition to offering RV and tent camping spots, most properties provide the option of staying in a small log cabin.

Many mold avoiders have reported that these cabins usually feel good to them in terms of toxic mold.

Mold generally does not grow on the logs.

In addition, because the furnishings are very basic, the cross-contamination potential may be much less than is present in a hotel.

Periodically after the wood is refinished, KOA cabins can be a problem in terms of triggering chemical reactivities.

In addition, pesticides are sometimes used in the cabins at some properties.

Checking with management to see whether chemicals have recently been used thus may be a good idea.

The mattresses for the beds in these cabins are made out of foam with a plastic cover.

This makes them easier to wash than a mattress covered in fabric would be.

Guests supply their own linens.

The cabins have electricity and a porch for sitting outside.

Many KOA's are located in places with good air quality, though checking with other mold avoiders about this is always important.

All KOA's have bathrooms with showers available to their guests.

Some of these bathrooms are fine in terms of mold while others are more problematic.

Although KOA's have automatic laundry facilities available to their guests, these may be very likely to be contaminated with particularly bad toxins.

Hand washing sheets, towels, clothing and other items is strongly suggested.

The main advantage of KOA's for the mold avoidance sabbatical is that they give many of the advantages of a camping experience but allow individuals to sleep inside on a bed.

This may be much more comfortable for people who have various sensitivities or who would not be comfortable sleeping on the ground.

Depending on the location, KOA cabins may be priced at anywhere from $50-75 per night. Discounts may be available for longer stays.

Simple cabins offered by other businesses possibly may be okay too, though it is impossible to say for sure unless a mold avoider has visited them.

Mercey Hot Springs (about two hours from the San Francisco Bay Area) offers simple one-room cabins that as of this writing have been reported as tolerable by a number of mold avoiders.

RV Camping

A non-toxic RV conceivably could be an excellent shelter for a mold avoidance sabbatical, since it would allow individuals to spend time in particularly pristine places while still having some of the comforts of home (such as sleeping indoors in a bed as well as having access to a kitchen, toilet and indoor shower).

Unfortunately, practically all RV's that are likely to be immediately available to those considering a mold avoidance sabbatical should be assumed to be problematic with regard to mold toxins or unacceptable chemical toxins.

Possibly a purchased cargo trailer could serve as a refuge for an avoidance sabbatical, allowing individuals to sleep inside.

Since the trailer could be used later on or sold, this could provide a relatively low-cost way for individuals to have more comfort on the sabbatical while staying in a more pristine place.

An off-gassed Camplite also likely would be a reliable choice for a sabbatical.

Otherwise, the use of RV's for the avoidance sabbatical is not suggested.

Tent Camping

Tent camping is a relatively reliable way for individuals to get clear of toxins that very often are problems in buildings or RV's.

In addition, tent camping may be done in many particularly good locations where hotels would not be available.

Another good thing about tent camping is that it encourages people to spend a higher percentage of their time outside in the fresh air rather than staying indoors.

A downside of tent camping is that individuals who are very sick and very reactive may have a difficult time with it.

Exposures to noise, light, campfire smoke and bugs can be particularly irritating to them.

Weather that is relatively hot or relatively cold may be intolerable for them.

Those with pain issues can find sleeping on the ground or on a camping cot to be uncomfortable.

Setting up the tent, cooking outdoors and doing other needed activities can feel overwhelming for those who are ill.

Another downside of tent camping is that purchasing the equipment needed for a sabbatical is likely to be relatively expensive.

Those planning to tent camp in most locations probably would be best off having a fallback plan to be able to sleep in their vehicle if the weather gets bad.

Desert wind can make sleeping in a tent impossible unless it is in a sheltered spot, and rain in other locations can make tent camping unpleasant.

Even though it may be a bit more difficult to set up, a larger tent - such as one with a screen room that can be used during the day - may be particularly appropriate for the mold avoidance sabbatical.

Camping in a place with a good shower and nearby restaurants or grocery stores also can make a tent camping sabbatical much easier.

Although the small amount of mold that may grow on a tent as a result of rain in a good location is likely to be non-toxic, the synthetic material of tents tends to be cross-contaminated easily.

It therefore is important to protect tents from exposures to suspicious buildings or outdoor areas.

Many new tents have cross-contamination from the factory, but generally this is only moderately problematic regular toxic mold.

Usually most of the problem can be addressed by rinsing the tent and letting it dry.

Tents should not be washed in automatic washers during the sabbatical since this has the potential of contaminating them with particularly problematic toxin.

Very occasionally, new tents are cross-contaminated with particularly problematic toxins.

This may be especially likely to happen when tents have been purchased and then returned by other customers.

Those individuals with chemical sensitivities may find it difficult to obtain any new tent that is tolerable for them.

Although the tent camping sabbatical has some disadvantages, a number of individuals have successfully started out their mold avoidance efforts in this way.

For those who can make the logistics work, it may be a very good choice.

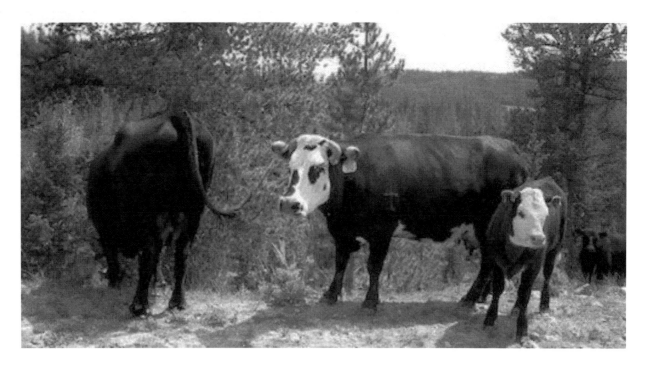

The mountains above Dubois (that's Du-boy), Wyoming.

Chapter 15

What About a Tent in the Backyard?

Not infrequently, individuals who suspect that their home has a problem with toxic mold are strongly inclined to see if they would feel better by getting out of the house and into a tent in their own backyard.

While this seems on the surface like a reasonable activity, a number of factors make it not work out very well most of the time.

First, insofar as super toxins are a problem in the outdoor air, moving outdoors may not be helpful at all.

It might even be worse than being inside the house.

If the house is contaminated with super toxins, some of them will get outside the house through the ventilation system.

Therefore, the backyard may have enough of those super toxins to feel just as problematic as the house.

If belongings are contaminated with super toxins, then using them for camping outside likely will prevent any progress from being made.

If the house is contaminated with super toxins, then going into the house (e.g. to use the bathroom or kitchen) without decontaminating afterwards very likely will totally ruin the experiment.

Even if the only problem in the house is cross-contaminated possessions from a previous bad residence, it has the potential of causing enough cross-contamination of people briefly entering the house to keep them from getting anywhere close to clear.

The one circumstance when the "tent in the backyard" approach might be expected to be helpful is when the house in question has a substantial problem with regular toxic mold but little or no super toxin involvement.

In that case, people might benefit from having their exposure to that regular toxic mold reduced from a very high amount to a much lower amount by getting out of the house and into a tent.

Whatever exposure to the regular toxic mold they got while in the tent (e.g. toxins sticking to clothing and hair when they used the house or toxins getting out of the house through the ventilation system) might not be a deal killer, if only regular toxic mold rather than super toxins is involved.

Of course, people who are trying to find out whether they are hyperreactive to toxic mold usually have no idea whether super toxins are playing a role in their illness.

That makes it hard to know whether the tent in the backyard experiment would be worth trying.

One thing to consider here is the anecdotal observation that people generally first get sick with chronic multisystem illness when they are being exposed to substantial amounts of super toxins either in their home or workplace.

That would suggest that if people are still living in the home where they got sick, and if they do not strongly suspect that a workplace rather than home exposure may have been primarily responsible for why they became sick, super toxins may be suspected as playing a role.

An additional consideration is that possessions will remain plenty toxic to keep people sick for quite a long time after they have been removed from an environment being affected by super toxins.

Certainly they may remain toxic -- and have the potential to cross-contaminate other objects or people -- for at least five years or more.

Therefore, insofar as a residence contains possessions transferred from a home or workplace where an individual became ill with chronic multisystem disease, super toxins should be suspected as playing a role.

Here are some real-world stories focused on people who have succeeded with the backyard camping experiment, along with some speculation with regard to why it may have worked for them when it does not help most people at all.

Example 1:

This individual became ill with ME/CFS during an outbreak. Over the next thirty years, she moved a number of times and recovered some of her health with apparently random relapses. She had been living in a particular house for a number of years with her partner, who showed no signs of illness. She became interested in the possibility that toxic mold might be playing a role in her illness and ran an ERMI test on the house, which came up high. Substantial amounts of mold were found hidden in the home. She benefited from moving into a tent in the backyard, entering the house only to use the kitchen and bathroom. She washed some of her possessions from the house and was not bothered by them. Her car also felt okay to her and later to other mold avoiders. When her partner did some remediation of the mold and moved all of their possessions into a back room of the house, it felt somewhat better to her, but not good enough that she wanted to live in it. Then when he moved all the possessions back into their usual places, she felt strongly suicidal.

Comments: In general, although this home had a substantial problem with regular toxic mold, it does not seem to have super toxins growing in it. Super toxins cannot be washed from belongings to the point that those items can be tolerated by severe responders, and they do not permit severe responders to live in a tent in the backyard but use the bathroom as needed. Usually there is at least some cross-contamination of vehicles as well. In addition, this person had been out of the environment in which she got sick for decades, and her partner was not sick. The suicidal response does suggest that one or more of their possessions was contaminated with a super toxin though, and this may have been a main factor driving her continued illness.

Example 2:

This individual become suddenly ill with severe ME/CFS while living in an area known for having particular problems with super toxins in the outdoor air and in many buildings. A number of years later, he moved into his parents' home in a different location, bringing with him only his personal possessions such as clothes and books. His parents suffered from respiratory complaints but no signs of multisystem illness. The house tested as being very problematic on the ERMI test and a mold problem was found. The individual purchased all new possessions and tried moving into a tent in the backyard, using the home only for bathroom and kitchen needs. He experienced improvements.

Comments: Again, this person did not get sick in this home and no one else got sick in it either. It certainly had a problem with regular toxic mold, but there is no indication of any super toxins being present except possibly on this individual's own possessions, which he put aside for this experiment and which were stored mostly in his own room rather than the kitchen or bathroom.

Example 3:

This individual became sick with multisystem illness while living in a home that came up as having large amounts of Wallemia on the ERMI, but she suspects that her workplace may have been even more of a problem. She retired from work but remained ill. She eventually moved without any of her old possessions into a Camplite RV, which she was able to live in successfully (recovering much of her health) parked on her own land next to her house. With effort, she was able to reclaim a few of her belongings from the house. She stated that while the mold in her house was problematic, she has run into other mold that seemed worse to her.

Comments: This story does not sound like substantial amounts of super toxins were present in this person's home. Items long exposed to super toxins are not generally remediable to the point where hyperreactive people can tolerate them. An alternative explanation is that super toxins in the workplace prompted her illness but that the substantial amount of regular toxic mold in her home affected her negatively once she was already ill.

Example 4:

This individual got suddenly ill with severe ME/CFS shortly after moving into what she immediately suspected was a problematic apartment. She recovered a large amount of her health within a few months of leaving the apartment, living in a different home without any of the possessions from the place where she got sick. Then when she moved her possessions into this new home, she became extremely sick again within just a few weeks. Suspecting that the house had become a problem, she tried moving into a tent in the backyard, using the house only for showering and bringing some possessions from the house with her. She felt a bit better, but it was nothing dramatic. Then, after going on a mold avoidance sabbatical, she returned to the house and found that it as well as all the objects from it were wholly intolerable to her. Few other buildings she visited bothered her nearly as much. She purchased all new possessions and set up a tent in the backyard, staying out of the house and decontaminating (showering and changing clothes) after the rare occasions when she had to go inside. She experienced substantial health gains.

Comments: This seems a clear case of possessions being cross-contaminated by super toxins in a bad home and then causing problems when brought to a different home. Since this person did well living in the current house before the contaminated possessions were brought in, a guess here is that the house itself was okay with regard to super toxins and that cross-contamination was the only issue with it. This may explain why she was able to do well living just outside the house; if the house itself had had super toxin contamination, that likely would not have been possible.

Again, these cases where people achieved benefits camping in their own backyard are exceptions. Many others have tried this and obtained no benefits whatsoever -- in many cases mistakenly convincing themselves for a time that mold probably had nothing to do with their illness after all.

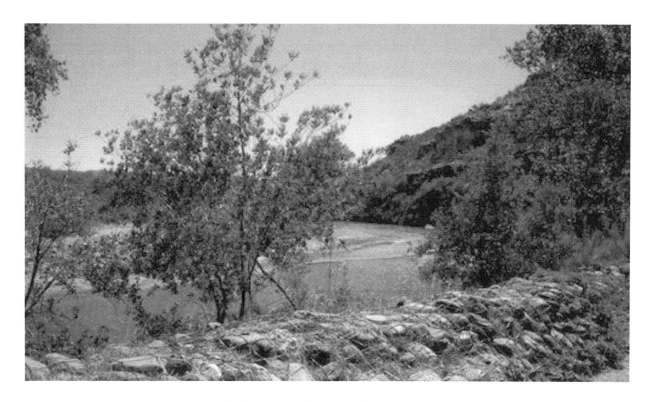

A river near Camp Verde, Arizona.

Chapter 16

The Return Home

People who succeed in getting fairly clear on the mold avoidance sabbatical report having a variety of experiences while away.

Some don't feel much different during the sabbatical.

Some actually feel worse in certain ways.

Some feel a bit better than they usually do.

A small minority of people report feeling much better or almost well.

One issue here is that when a very toxic body gets relatively clear of exposures, it may start to dump toxins at a rapid clip.

This can result in feeling worse, often with many of the same symptoms of exposures.

Hints of Getting Clear

A few specific symptoms tend to be associated with getting clear and detoxing more than being in a bad place.

Sleep tends to be sounder in a clear place, with patients often reporting sleeping very deeply or having less need for sleep medications.

Increased sensitivities to objects (including ones brought from home), to buildings, to pollution or to household chemicals may occur.

Sometimes the body will spontaneously sweat much more.

Exercise intolerance or activity intolerance may go down.

There thus may be clues that the experiment is going well, even during the sabbatical.

After the Sabbatical

The most important outcome of the sabbatical occurs after it is over, when the individual returns to the home environment and considers whether it triggers a negative effect.

In some cases, a reaction may happen immediately upon return to the usual environment.

In other cases, and especially with certain toxins, a delay of up to 12-36 hours may occur between exposure and emergence of noticeable symptoms.

In many cases, emergence of symptoms after return from the avoidance sabbatical is dramatic.

This is not something where people have to guess whether they are being affected.

If hyperreactivity is present and the sabbatical was done in the proper way, symptoms will emerge and further exposure will feel intolerable within a relatively short period of time.

An important consideration here is not to ignore mood shifts.

Feelings of depression, suicidal ideation, anxiety, panic, irritability, anger or other negative emotions frequently emerge with re-exposures to problem substances after return from an avoidance sabbatical.

Next Steps

After a successful sabbatical, the general goal is to make environmental changes with regard to identified exposures (such as from buildings, locations or objects) to try to reduce the reactions.

This almost always becomes easier over time, as people become more experienced and stay clear of the worst toxins for a longer periods of time.

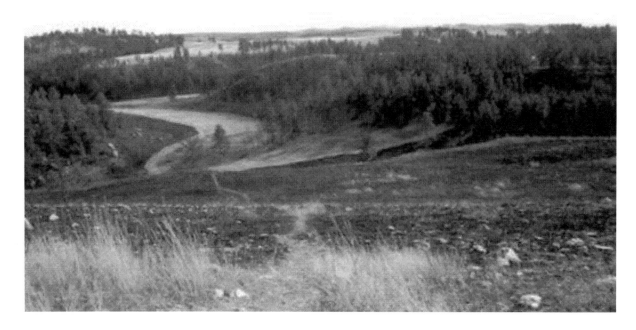

The Black Hills of South Dakota.

Chapter 17

A Sabbatical Alternative

On occasion, individuals with chronic multisystem disease express interest in pursuing mold avoidance without starting out with an avoidance sabbatical.

In some cases, these individuals say that they already know that they are reactive to their environment and just want to get away from it.

Other individuals have limited financial or physical resources and don't feel that they will have enough left over after doing a sabbatical to pursue avoidance successfully.

Misconceptions

In many cases, those without much knowledge about mold avoidance believe that if they merely move from their problematic home to a better one, in their same community, they should be able to make significant health gains.

Unfortunately, for people with chronic multisystem illness, that very often is not what happens.

Insofar as these individuals continue to get any exposure whatsoever to super toxins - from contaminated possessions, visits to particularly problematic buildings or just the outside air - they likely will continue to feel just as sick as they did when they were living in the particularly problematic building.

Whether it is worth it in the long run for an individual to move out of a home that is particularly problematic with regard to super toxins without leaving contaminated possessions behind is an open question.

It could be that even if hyperreactive people do not feel any better after the move, they might have continued to decline at a core level if they had continued to be exposed to a greater quantity of the toxins in question over subsequent months or years.

In addition, insofar as contaminated possessions eventually die down enough to be tolerated, individuals might then "spontaneously" regain some of their health.

Regardless, most people who are considering pursuing avoidance say they are doing so with the hope of making health gains in the near future, rather than merely to keep from declining or to feel better five or ten years down the road.

Based on the case studies seen so far, this only will happen for hyperreactive individuals if they successfully manage to avoid exposure to even small amounts of super toxins (as well as substantial amounts of regular mold toxins).

Skipping the Sabbatical

The general idea here is to follow the instructions for setting up the avoidance sabbatical, except with the intention of going forward with it permanently.

It thus involves the same difficulties as the avoidance sabbatical.

Especially when people are very ill or have limited resources - and when they feel confident that their current environment is very problematic for them - it may be an option worth considering.

However, moving from a problematic environment to a different one without first making any attempt to get clear always will have an element of risk to it.

There always will be some chance that the new environment will be problematic and therefore that no progress will be achieved.

For those who want to give it a try, following these steps may increase the likelihood that the move will result in health improvements.

1. Consider the comments that other mold avoiders have made about the locations being considered.

If a location is suspected as being particularly problematic (especially with regard to outdoor super toxins), then it probably should not be considered an acceptable choice for someone who is trying to make improvements without getting clear first.

Mold avoiders tend to have a much easier time and make much more progress in areas where the air is particularly good.

Insofar as the option is available, choosing a location that is excellent rather than just okay in terms of the outdoor air may be a good idea.

2. Consider available housing options carefully.

Preferably, housing options would be evaluated by someone experienced in mold avoidance or with an ERMI test.

That is not always feasible though.

Homes where current residents seem wholly healthy may be less risky choices than ones where residents are experiencing any sort of "mystery disease" (including emotional issues).

Homes where people have become mostly or fully recovered from chronic multisystem illness generally seem to work well for others as well.

However, it is not necessarily advisable for people with this sort of illness to live together, due to possible effects of toxins (including those that might be cross-contaminating possessions as well as those that might be excreted via detox) as well as the possibility of transmission of active infections particularly associated with this sort of illness.

Some people moving from a particularly problematic environment have gotten off to a successful start just choosing a home sight unseen in a different location and moving there without any of their contaminated belongings.

The hope here is that a random building will be good enough to give people a start at making some health progress and thus to be more able to seek out better options in the future.

A key point is to not sign any sort of long-term lease and not to buy many new possessions, since if the randomly chosen home turns out to be bad then neither it nor the possessions that have been kept in it may be usable in the future.

3. Take no possessions.

Since it's impossible for someone who has not yet become clear to determine how problematic possessions might be, not taking anything is the safest course.

In some cases, just a single possession contaminated with particularly problematic toxins can prevent any progress from occurring.

Possessions from the suspect environment may be put into storage for consideration later on, donated to others, or discarded.

At minimum, any possessions that are transferred to the new residence should be washed and then kept separate so that people will be more likely to be able to tell if they are having a negative effect.

If possessions cannot be washed, then they definitely should not be brought along since they will have the potential of cross-contaminating everything else.

4. Logistics

The idea of moving in this way is to follow the basic concepts of the avoidance sabbatical, except on a permanent rather than temporary basis.

Following the logistics suggestions with regard to the mold avoidance sabbatical may yield the best results.

Part 3

PURSUING AVOIDANCE

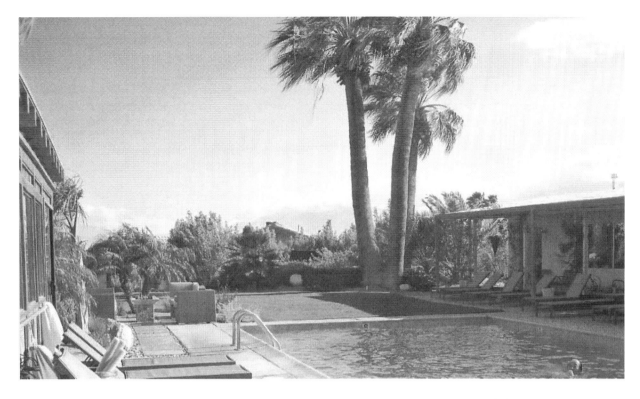

A hot springs resort called The Spring in Desert Hot Springs, California.

Chapter 18

After The Sabbatical

Insofar as people realize subsequent to a mold avoidance sabbatical that they are reacting negatively to their usual environment, the next step is to organize life in a different and better environment.

In a small minority of cases, people discover that their current homes are relatively okay for them and that they are being negatively affected primarily by a few cross-contaminated possessions or by personal cross-contaminations as a result of visiting other problematic environments.

In those cases, attending to those cross-contaminations may provide health gains without the need to move elsewhere.

In some other cases, the primary issue turns out to be many possessions cross-contaminated elsewhere (such as in a previous residence) with a particularly problematic toxin.

In that case, removing all the possessions from the home and cleaning it thoroughly may or may not be enough to make the dwelling tolerable.

Unfortunately, many individuals with chronic multisystem illness come back from the mold avoidance sabbatical to find that their home is problematic to the point of not being livable for them - due to mold growing in the building itself, to the whole location being a problem, or to cross-contamination that lingers even after attempts are made to address it.

At that point, most people tend to focus their attention on achieving three major goals.

1. Deciding what to do about possessions.

Depending on the level of reactivity and the particular toxins involved, in some cases it may be possible to clean some or all possessions well enough to have them not prompt reactions.

If this is not the case, then they will need to be put in storage or disposed of in some other way.

2. Finding a more tolerable place to live.

This could be a house, apartment, hotel, vehicle or tent. Those who make the most successful recoveries tend to consider location effects as well.

3. Gaining support of others.

Making others understand that hyperreactivity is a real phenomenon and that mold avoidance has the potential to be helpful enough to make it worthwhile can be a challenge.

Insofar as support can be obtained, it may make the subsequent journey easier.

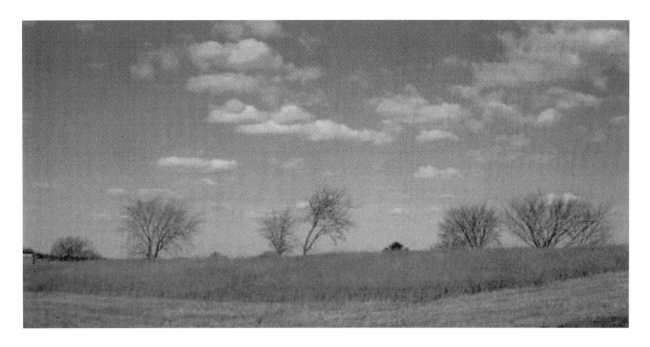

Southwestern Minnesota.

Chapter 19

Dealing with Possessions

Possessions contaminated with super toxins may not be able to be cleaned to the point that those who are hyperreactive to toxic mold can tolerate them without ill effects.

This may be the case regardless of whether the source of the cross-contamination is the home itself, the outdoor air, or another cross-contaminated item.

In other cases, contaminated items may be able to be cleaned to the point that the hyperreactive individual is able to tolerate them.

The only way to know what kind of an effect that possessions might be having and whether they can be cleaned sufficiently not to have any effect is to get really clear first.

Therefore, in the early stages of mold avoidance, proceeding very cautiously with regard to concluding that particular items are okay may be a good idea.

Proceeding Cautiously

Insofar as items have been exposed to a problematic environment, washing them (or at least wiping them with a damp cloth) is a good idea.

This will remove the spores and spore fragments, thus decreasing their cross-contamination potential substantially.

The next step is to put the items aside for a bit, to give them a chance to off-gas away from the problematic environment.

They then may be approached carefully, to see if they prompt reactions.

A challenge here is that even after a successful avoidance sabbatical, many people are not fully unmasked.

As a result, they may not be able to accurately detect the presence of toxins that will be problematic for them as well as they will be able to subsequent to additional avoidance.

Being conservative in terms of which possessions are reclaimed early in avoidance thus may be in order.

For instance, it may be better to put everything that would be nice to reclaim into storage for a while, and then to return to it when confidence about the ability to identify problem toxins becomes higher.

Another approach is to reclaim just a few washed items at the beginning, with the goal of considering whether they seem to be causing any issues.

Additional Thoughts

A few more comments on reclaiming items.

1. Items that will be in close contact with a hyperreactive individual (such as clothes or bedding) may be less desirable to reclaim since they will have more of an effect.

2. Needed papers are a problem for many people. Photocopying or scanning them when possible may be a better idea than holding on to the originals.

3. Toxins seem to stick particularly well to synthetic materials (including plastic) and to fibers. Other types of items (especially metal) may be more likely to be successfully reclaimed.

4. Items that were exposed to the environment where the person first became sick with chronic multisystem disease often are contaminated with super toxins and thus may be especially difficult to remediate.

5. Items that trigger strong burning or itching sensations may be contaminated with what has been called the Hell Toxin and should be handled with extreme care, especially in terms of their cross-contamination potential. See Chapter 31.

6. Items that have been only briefly exposed to a problematic environment tend to be much easier to remediate than items exposed to problematic environments for an extended period of time.

7. A frequent question from people starting out is whether it is okay to keep their computer equipment in the early stages of avoidance, since this is expensive to replace. Unless the computer is contaminated with the Hell Toxin, reports are that this is not usually disastrous. Of course, the computer should be wiped with a damp cloth to remove dust and (if a laptop) put into a new case. While contaminated computers might well cause a reaction when being used, computers have not been observed to cross-contaminate other possessions very much. The exception is when they are contaminated with the Hell Toxin, in which case they have the potential of irreparably cross-contaminating all other possessions in the environment (especially when the fan goes on).

8. Another frequent question from people starting out with avoidance is whether they need to replace their cars. Insofar as the Hell Toxin is a factor in the illness, that would be wise. In addition, cars that have been kept in locations that have a substantial problem with the outdoor Mystery Toxin (see Chapter 30) may not die down for many years and thus may be worthwhile to replace. However, some mold avoiders using scrupulous decontamination techniques have managed to continue using their current cars for at least a while after moving from problem homes, even when certain super toxins have been involved.

9. If items do not feel good enough to be used after washing, it is possible that other remediation techniques will improve them enough to make them tolerable. See Chapter 37 for a discussion of remediating cross-contaminations.

Sorting

People who are unmasked enough to determine whether possessions are okay may not want to spend much time sorting through those possessions in order to effectively put them into storage or to dispose of them.

Asking or hiring a less reactive person to help with the work may be a good idea.

Some people have put work into sorting through their possessions before going on a sabbatical or moving, because they fear that intensification response will make it difficult for them to get near those objects later on.

A downside to this approach is that the sorting can take quite a long time if energy and cognitive focus are low.

Storage

Items that are not immediately reclaimable may eventually improve enough to be tolerated, and so putting especially cherished possessions into storage may be worth considering.

It probably would be preferable to wash items (or at least wipe them with a damp cloth) before putting them into storage, in order to remove mold spores from them.

Mold spores contaminating possessions may have the ability to start new colonies, and this is to be avoided when the mold in question has demonstrated itself to be particularly problematic.

The denaturing of mold toxins seems to occur through evaporation.

Therefore, leaving items relatively exposed (rather than wrapping them in plastic) may be a good idea.

Heat and dry air possibly may help items to denature faster.

Reports suggest that possessions contaminated with super toxins may take at least five years or more to die down to the point that a hyperreactive person can reclaim them.

In some cases, substantially more time may be needed.

Possibly ozoning items may decrease the amount of time needed for items to die down, even if the ozoning does not resolve the problem immediately.

Some reports suggest that items that have been stored in certain locations have become worse over time, at least in some cases as a result of new mold growth.

Disposal

In cases when particularly bad toxins are involved, some individuals disposing of their possessions have decided to dump everything to reduce the likelihood that others will be harmed by those toxins.

This especially has been the case when the toxins involved seem unusual in some way, such as Hell Toxin.

Other people have argued that many of these particularly bad toxins are common in the environment, that small quantities do not seem harmful to healthy individuals, and that the toxins eventually will denature to the point that they are not a problem.

Those taking this position often choose to sell or donate their possessions rather than discarding them.

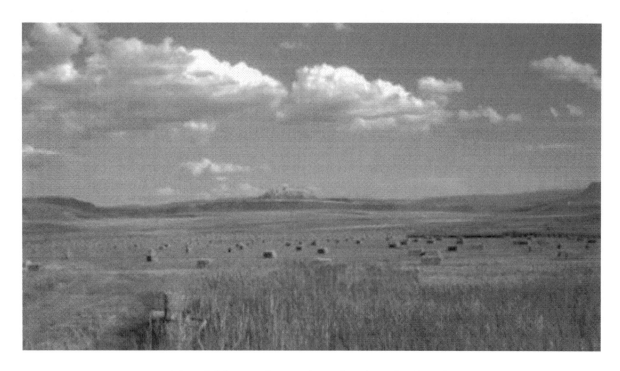

A hayfield near the northern border of Colorado.

Chapter 20

Avoidance Over Time

People who commit themselves to pursuing avoidance often assume that their first order of business is to find a new home that is clear enough for them and to settle down there for the indefinite future.

A minority of people with moderate or severe chronic multisystem disease do accomplish this goal.

Especially if someone has been living in a particularly problematic place and is only moderately sick, their hyperreactivity may be low enough for them to tolerate some available residences and to start to move toward wellness in them.

In many cases, however, things do not work out this way.

What is much more typical is for people to believe or hope that a particular home will be good enough, only to conclude at some point in the future (days or months later) that it is having a negative effect.

Starting Out

Finding a home that will be good enough for someone who is very hyperreactive to do well in permanently is usually a real challenge.

The small amounts of regular toxic mold present in the vast majority of buildings may be too much for hyperreactive individuals to handle without negative effects.

Even after a successful two-week avoidance sabbatical, people may not be clear enough to identify immediately all toxins that will be problematic for them.

It can take a while longer to become clear enough and skilled enough to do that.

In addition, very rarely have individuals who are moderately or severely affected with chronic multisystem illness started out with avoidance by living in a tent or an RV on a full-time basis.

The logistics of doing this tend to be too difficult for people to manage when they are still really sick and feeling overwhelmed.

Therefore, it often seems to work out best when people consider the first 6-12 months of avoidance as an interim stage rather than as one where the goal is to make permanent decisions about living situations.

A Temporary Home

For almost everyone who started out as moderately severely or severely affected, finding a house or apartment that is good enough to be tolerated without noticeable negative effects has been a first step in the avoidance process.

A residence that is reasonably good with regard to all types of exposures (indoor toxins, outdoor toxins and cross-contamination) will give the system a chance to calm down and to start repairing itself.

Such a place generally provides some improvements in symptoms fairly quickly, with additional improvements gradually accumulating over a period of months.

However, in many cases, people eventually conclude that the place that they thought was good enough at the beginning actually is not nearly as good as they need in order to keep making progress.

At that point, they may start looking for something better -- either a different building or a camping lifestyle.

Some Suggestions

Buildings that feel okay early in avoidance can reveal themselves to be over tolerance later on or can actually go bad.

Therefore, refraining from signing any long-term commitments such as long-term leases can be important.

Certainly, unless it is certain that it can be resold at a good price, purchasing a home should be avoided at this stage.

In general, people who make the most gains with avoidance tend to do their best to get clear as much as possible even if they are living in a non-pristine place.

For instance, they may spend a great deal of time outdoors in place with particularly good air or sleep outdoors as often as they can.

Getting clear on a frequent basis may make a non-pristine house seem more bothersome.

However, it is still recommended, since it also will promote increased feelings of health and ability to do more.

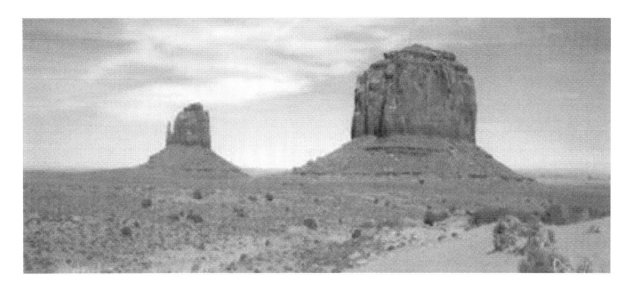

Monument Valley Navajo Tribal Park in northeastern Arizona.

Chapter 21

Evaluating Residences

Almost all modern buildings have enough regular toxic mold in them to have a negative effect on some hyperreactive individuals.

In addition, people who are pursuing avoidance may find that their own ability to live amongst particular toxins changes over time.

For instance, many people find that their tendency to be bothered by toxins increases substantially during the first few months or years of avoidance as they become increasingly clear on a regular basis and thus feel increasingly good.

(Often at some point later in their recovery, their reactivity goes back down again without their losing their health gains.)

Moreover, even if buildings have no mold actually growing in them, individuals still may be negatively affected by being in a bad location or by being cross-contaminated with particularly bad toxins.

Therefore, the idea that there is such a thing as "mold-safe" or "mold-free" housing may be a bit optimistic.

With few exceptions, there only is housing that is good enough for a particular person to tolerate at a particular point in time, rather than housing that is excellent enough to be tolerable by everyone.

An important question thus is how to find that "good-enough" housing.

Tolerance Testing

Once people have become clear enough to be able to gauge their reactions to environments, they almost always agree that the most accurate way for them to determine whether a building is good enough for them is to spend time in it.

Preferably this would be an extended period of time.

For instance, spending at least one night in a potential home before making any kind of commitment is a good idea, especially for people just starting out.

Spending a couple of weeks would be even better.

Visiting the potential residence during different weather conditions also may be helpful.

In some cases, factors like rain or wind direction may cause particularly problematic toxins to become apparent at certain times.

In most cases, mold toxins tend to fall downwards and accumulate on horizontal surfaces.

Therefore, testing a residence by lying face-down on the floor and breathing in may be more effective than standing upright.

Mood shifts are an important clue with regard to determining whether a home is problematic.

If a building triggers depression, anxiety, suicidal ideation or other negative feelings, that is an important sign that it is not a good-enough place.

The ability to sleep deeply in a building is a positive sign that it is good enough.

Non-refreshing half-sleep or inability to sleep very often is associated with inflammation prompted by unacceptable amounts of mold toxins.

Emergence of any other negative physical or cognitive symptoms may be taken to suggest that the building may be problematic as well.

Some mold avoiders state that ultimately, learning to listen to their intuition has been helpful in allowing them to quickly evaluate whether an environment is okay for them, even before any concrete symptoms emerge.

This does tend to take some practice to develop, however.

ERMI Testing

For mold avoiders who are not yet confident in their ability to determine whether buildings are okay for them, the ERMI test (described in Chapter 53) may serve as an adjunct to their own perceptions.

The ERMI test does have limitations though.

In some cases, ERMI tests can miss the presence even of large amounts of problematic mold (such as when the spores are sealed tightly inside a wall).

The ERMI also does not have the ability to identify super toxins present in an environment.

It is looking only at the molds species that are present, and those molds often have the potential of making a variety of toxins depending on the circumstances.

In addition, ERMI scores have a confidence interval of +/- 3 points.

This means that if, for instance, a building is rated as a 0, the actual score could be anywhere from -3 to +3.

In short, just because the ERMI suggests that a building is good does not mean that it is going to be tolerable for any particular individual.

However, the ERMI may be successful in helping to eliminate buildings that are particularly problematic when mold avoiders are not very experienced.

Building Types

On average, traditional building styles often may have more potential to be acceptable with regard to toxic mold than modern building styles.

Any home without wall insulation or drywall may have the potential of being less problematic.

Often buildings such as log homes, adobe homes, cement block homes, metal homes or straw bale homes qualify, for instance.

Homes that have been poorly maintained or that have sat empty for an extended period of time may be more problematic, on average.

Homes that have experienced flooding usually have toxic mold problems.

Unfortunately, though, it is very difficult to predict with any confidence which homes might have mold in them based on building characteristics.

Pretty much any building could be problematic for those hyperreactive to mold toxins.

Commitments

In general, avoiding commitments when it comes to housing usually is a smart idea for mold avoiders.

It is very difficult to ensure that any home will remain good into the future.

The possibility that the outdoor air in a particular location will not remain okay adds another layer of risk to the equation.

People who are just starting out with avoidance may find that their reactivity changes over time.

They also may become choosier as time goes on with regard to the type of housing that they are willing to accept.

Therefore, signing a long-term lease or buying a home is generally something that should be avoided.

Some options that have worked for mold avoiders include:

1. Signing a shorter lease (such as 1-3 months) and possibly paying a higher amount per month.

2. Negotiating an agreement that the lease can be broken with a doctor's note that moving out of the building is a health requirement.

3. Putting plans in place to sublet the rental if it does not work out.

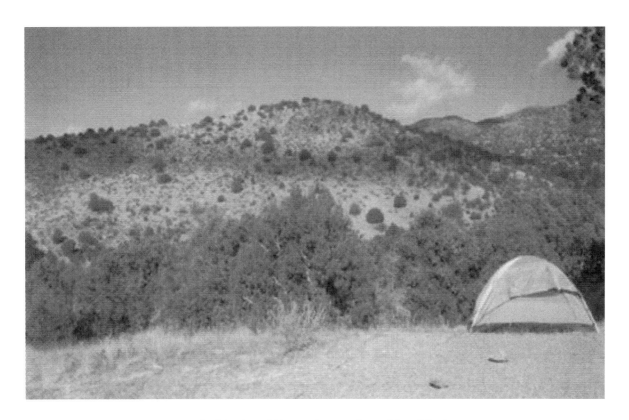

Lincoln National Forest in southern New Mexico.

Chapter 22

Tent Camping

Getting clear by camping in a good area has the potential of facilitating improvements that will allow people to be less reactive, to sleep well in places that they previously would have found to be uncomfortable, and to feel more energetic.

There is absolutely no guarantee that this will happen right away on a camping trip, however.

In the meantime, people who are very ill may have a hard time tent camping.

Reactivities to noise, light and wood smoke may present particular problems for them.

Some have difficulties sleeping in anything other than a conventional bed.

Temperature regulation problems may make camping especially uncomfortable.

The level of activity needed to successfully camp may be far more than some people are able to handle while still very sick.

However, once people have made some good improvements, they may find camping a beneficial experience with a variety of positive attributes.

Since the vast majority of buildings have enough mold toxin in them to prompt reactions, tent camping may be one of the few opportunities for very hyperreactive people to really get clear.

Tent camping also has the potential of allowing people to spend more time in areas where the air is particularly good.

In addition, tent camping allows people to try out different locations while sleeping in the same shelter, thereby giving them more of a sense of the extent to which outdoor locations make a difference for them.

Getting Started

Many mold avoiders have never previously camped and feel overwhelmed by the whole idea.

As a first step, reading about camping gear and visiting a camping store to take a look at the equipment available may create some level of comfort.

REI employees tend to be particularly good at helping new campers learn about products that might be suitable for them.

Once equipment is purchased, it may be a good idea to try sleeping in the tent in the backyard of a good home or on an overnight trip before going on a longer trip.

This may allow people to start to feel comfortable with their camping equipment and to get used to sleeping outdoors.

A downside to this sort of overnight trip is that if the air quality is not very good in the area, people may not feel any better sleeping in a tent than they do in a reasonably good home.

In some cases they might even feel worse, since there may be less protection from the outdoor toxins when sleeping in a tent.

In order to understand the appeal of camping, making a special effort to go on a trip to a location where the air has been reported to be excellent may be worthwhile.

For many people, realizing what a difference good air quality can make provides a very good incentive to seek it out more in the future.

Extended Camping

Although it is not for everyone, tent camping for a longer period of time may be worth considering.

Many mold avoiders credit spending substantial amounts of time camping in the wilderness with helping them to move toward recovery and to reduce their mold reactivity more quickly.

Anecdotal reports suggest that getting clear enough for inflammation to move toward normal may be essential for achieving detoxification, addressing pathogens and promoting overall healing.

Many individuals are so hyperreactive that it is difficult for them to get clear enough to accomplish these goals unless they are in the wilderness.

Possibly, if people spend significant amounts of time in a really clear place on the front end of their avoidance experiences, their reactivity eventually may go down substantially.

This may mean that they will continue to do well even without such extreme avoidance later on.

Traveling Around

Insofar as mold avoiders have the ability to do so, traveling around while camping rather than staying in one place can be very informative in terms of the extent to which different locations have an effect on their feelings of well-being.

Traveling while camping takes somewhat more effort than staying one place, but the learning experience of trying out different locations may make it worthwhile.

In addition, when viewed with a spirit of wanting to have fun and pursue adventure, traveling around has the potential of being much more interesting and inspiring than remaining in one place.

For mold avoiders who have tried camping and not found it as helpful as they had hoped, spending some time traveling around may be especially beneficial.

Hopefully by trying out different locations, eventually people in this situation will hit upon one that feels good to them.

Seeking Shelter

Although one of the main goals in camping is to spend as much time as possible in the fresh air, most mold avoiders find that they do not end up spending every single night in a tent even on a short trip.

Weather conditions periodically may be inappropriate for tent camping.

Wind (which can be very strong in desert locations) is a particular enemy of tents, but rain also can be unpleasant.

Having a vehicle to sleep in comfortably when necessary can make camping much more enjoyable and manageable.

For instance, this could be an SUV (with the back seat folded down), the back of a pickup truck (with a camper shell on top), the back of a van, or a bench seat long enough to stretch out on.

One problem is that camping gear and other possessions have the potential of taking up much of the space in the vehicle, leaving little or no room for sleeping.

Storing most or all possessions in plastic bins that can be stacked outside when necessary (perhaps covered with a tarp) is one solution.

Towing a small cargo trailer to carry belongings also could be considered.

Many mold avoiders camping for extended periods of time periodically spend one or more nights in a hotel or the home of a friend.

Although it's rare for buildings to feel as good as sleeping outdoors in a good location, the taste of civilization can make occasional or frequent indoor stays feel worthwhile.

KOA cabins tend to be reviewed well by mold avoiders with regard to mold and therefore may be another option for tent campers looking to spend some time indoors.

Traveling Logistics

Those mold avoiders choosing to travel around while camping often select a particular destination point.

Then, taking into consideration factors such as anticipated air quality and desirable attractions, they map out a rough itinerary to get there.

However, it may be better not to make most plans too firm since locations have the potential of having problematic air quality even if they have been okay in the past.

For the most part, in the camping world, there is no such thing as a refund.

Therefore, it may be a better idea to wait until getting to the destination to pay for camping rather than making a reservation in advance.

Since some locations can unexpectedly reveal themselves to be problematic, paying for one night of camping at a time may be a good idea unless a significant discount can be obtained for a longer stay.

Although not everyone with mold reactivity is a morning person, it may be preferable to plan to arrive at each destination relatively early in the day (or at least a few hours before nightfall).

This will provide a better chance of getting a spot at campgrounds that will fill up, as well as allowing more time to pursue an alternative if things do not work out at the original destination.

Planning to stay in less popular locations during busy weekends or on holidays is another possible strategy.

Public Campgrounds

Public campgrounds (such as those that are part of state or national parks) usually provide basic accommodations for a modest fee (often $10-20 per night).

Campsites usually include a picnic table, a place to pitch the tent, and space for one or more vehicles.

Fire pits and barbecue grills are often present at the site.

In desert locations, sometimes a shade shelter is provided.

Water at public campgrounds may be available either at the campsite or in a common location.

Pit toilets or flush toilets are almost always available.

Rarely do national parks have shower facilities available for campers, but some state parks do.

Electricity is sometimes available at tent campsites for an extra fee, particularly in state parks.

Electric outlets where devices can be charged by campers also can be found in some campgrounds.

Private Campgrounds

Kampgrounds of America (KOA) and other private campgrounds frequently offer tent camping.

Prices tend to be more expensive (such as $20 or more per night).

Electricity at the site is often an option at commercial campgrounds.

Campsites at private campgrounds usually include a picnic table, charcoal grill, fire pit and water supply.

Most private campgrounds provide bathrooms with showers to their guests.

Sometimes these bathrooms may have mold problems or chemical issues, however.

Many private campgrounds and some public campgrounds have a designated outdoor sink for washing dishes.

Dispersed Camping

Dispersed camping is done on uncivilized lands, away from civilization.

The Bureau of Land Management (BLM) offers free dispersed camping on much of its land.

Some national parks and a few state parks allow dispersed camping as well.

When allowed, BLM camping is limited to 14 days in a 28 period within a 30-mile radius.

BLM does not currently require registration for dispersed camping, but national and state parks may.

The lack of water for dispersed camping necessitates bringing along a water supply.

The lack of toilets necessitates bringing along a small shovel to dig 6" deep cat holes to bury feces.

Although it may seem like a main attraction of dispersed camping is that it is free, many people also enjoy the feeling of being totally away from other people in the wilderness.

Bathing

A challenge when camping is keeping clean, with regard to dirt and sweat as well as toxins.

Unexpected cross-contaminations may require immediate washing up.

Some people (especially in the early stages of recovery) may find themselves unexpectedly covered with toxic sweat that seems imperative to wash off quickly as well.

Private campgrounds such as KOA's as well as some public campgrounds may have showers available, but those avoiding mold may not find all of these usable due to the presence of mold toxins or chemicals within.

If a bathroom is only moderately problematic, one alternative may be to use it to shower and then do a mini-decontamination (i.e. change clothes, rinse hair with water, wipe off face and neck with a wet cloth) afterwards.

Insofar as mold is not an issue and they are in a good location, hot springs often have pretty good shower facilities.

Large travel center chains (such as TravelCenters of America, Pilot and Love's) almost always have showers, and those showers have been reported to rarely have mold problems.

However, for those not purchasing large amounts of fuel for semi-trucks, the cost of a shower at a travel center is fairly expensive (e.g. $10-12).

Reportedly in most cases, no one objects if two people use the shower room at once for that price.

Truckers often accumulate extra shower passes and conceivably could be persuaded to give up one for a more reasonable sum.

If the weather is warm enough, bathing outdoors or in a tent may be an option.

Camping gear useful for getting clean outdoors is discussed in Chapter 23.

Mold Growth

Especially for those camping in humid and non-pristine areas, camping equipment or other possessions may be subject to bothersome mold growth.

Some individuals have reported that ozoning tents and other possessions on a regular basis (even every several days) can be helpful in keeping this in check.

Camping Safety

One concern about either tent camping or RV camping is physical safety.

This may include guarding against threats from humans, from animals, from plants and from accidents.

Women traveling alone tend to feel especially concerned about safety issues at first.

However, women who have spent extensive periods of time camping on their own in the US (whether for mold avoidance or for other reasons) usually report that they have felt surprisingly safe while doing so.

The camping culture tends to be protective of women camping alone, and so setting up within shouting distance of other campers may provide some added feelings of security.

Campgrounds that are within easy driving distance of metropolitan areas and that allow day use may use have the potential of attracting people who are rowdier or seem less trustworthy.

Camping in certain other countries (such as Mexico) may be much more dangerous with regard to threats from other people.

Desert camping often involves being wary of a variety of different poisonous creatures, including snakes, spiders and scorpions.

These animals tend to be more active during the night during the summer months.

Becoming knowledgeable about their behavior - and making preparations not to have to leave the tent at night (such as by having a "chamber pot" at the ready) - may be worth considering when camping in areas where they are present.

Mountain lions are present in some parts of the US but are said to be dangerous only to young children.

Bears are present in many wilderness areas in the US.

Only rarely do bears attack humans, but they may be attracted to their food.

Typical advice to avoid attracting bears includes not ever eating in the tent, storing food and garbage in the vehicle, and keeping the campsite free of food scraps.

Female bears who are separated from their cubs may attack, so that is something to be wary about.

Ticks (which can carry Lyme disease or a variety of other diseases) may be a threat in many camping areas.

Reading up on prevention suggestions and setting up away from high grass may be a good idea when camping in tick-endemic areas.

Valley Fever (a fungal infection spread by dirt blowing on the wind) may be a concern in certain desert areas (including southern Arizona and the Central Valley of California).

Learning to identify dangerous plants such as poison oak and poison ivy is a good idea.

Likely the biggest threat to campers is accidents.

Being careful is important.

When hiking, bringing along hiking poles (especially if poor coordination is an issue) and a whistle (to use if necessary to attract help) may be worthwhile.

Campgrounds often are filled with hazards such as uneven ground or tree limbs.

Always using a light and being especially careful after dark is a good idea.

Those experienced with firearms may consider bringing a gun with them (by far the most frequent reported use is shooting rattlesnakes).

Plenty of people camp successfully without a gun, however.

Letting someone know the planned itinerary and periodically checking in with that person for safety reasons could be considered.

Resources

The book series <u>The Best in Tent Camping</u> (available in paperback and Kindle formats) lists a variety of scenic campgrounds appropriate for camping in a small RV as well as a tent.

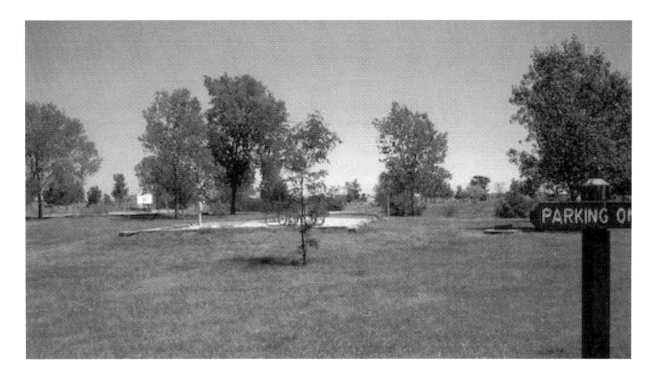

A campsite priced at less than $10/night at a state park in Kansas.

Chapter 23

Camping Gear

Appropriate equipment can lead to a camping experience that feels like less of a sacrifice with regard to being away from the comforts of civilization.

A downside is that camping gear has the potential of filling up even a large SUV, making sleeping in the back of the car less feasible.

Equipment also can be costly.

Especially for people who are just starting out with mold avoidance, return policies are very important.

Both REI (for members) and LL Bean allow products to be returned even after they have been washed or used.

People who have been camping for a while tend to develop their own preferences with regard to gear.

For novices who are considering camping for mold avoidance purposes, here are some thoughts.

Tents

Finding a tolerable tent is particularly important and often a challenge with regard to pursuing avoidance.

Tents are almost always made of "modern" materials that often are difficult for people with chemical sensitivities to tolerate right away.

At this writing, almost all of them have been treated with fire retardants as well.

In addition, tents may be cross-contaminated with mold toxins (from the factory, from the warehouse, from the store, from people who purchased and then returned them, or from being stored or used in a bad place).

Frequently the materials used to make tents can be particularly difficult to remediate.

Likely the only way to know for sure if a tent is going to be problematic is to rinse it and try sleeping in it -- which means that purchasing tents from a store that will take things back after they have been washed is important.

People who are very hyperreactive and very clear sometimes may find it difficult to find any tents that do not prompt any reactions, even after the tents are washed.

Letting the tent sit in the sun for a few days or a few weeks may be helpful in making it usable.

Particularly for those who are very reactive, having multiple tents on hand might be a good idea, to guard against the possibility that the tent will become unusable due to being cross-contaminated or destroyed by the wind.

Choosing a tent with substantial air flow (such as the liberal use of mesh) can be helpful with regard to creating a clear sleeping experience.

Once people get out into the wilderness, they often start to expel substantial amounts of toxins in their breath.

In a tent that doesn't have good air circulation, those toxins will be re-inhaled back into the system.

A few mold avoiders have reported having problems with mold growth underneath the bottom of their tents, with their solution being cutting the bottom out of the tent and sleeping on a cot.

Two-person tents (really suitable for just one person) tend to be very easy to put up and take down.

Most also can be used for backpacking trips.

However, two-person tents don't have much room and are most appropriate for people who intend to be outside of the tent except for when they are actually sleeping in it.

Since two-person tents don't take up much space in the car, having one on hand for emergencies (such as an after-dark arrival at a campsite or as a backup) could be a good idea.

Four-person tents allow enough space for two people to sleep reasonably comfortably, if they are planning to spend most of the rest of the time outside the tent.

For one person, a four-person tent provides some extra room that could be used for a low table or chair.

A tent with a screen room can provide a substantial amount of functionality for people who want to get work done at the campsite.

A screen room tent provides some protection from wind, rain and bugs, plus the shade makes using a laptop computer much more feasible.

A full-size screen room may be helpful in places where mosquitoes or other problematic insects are present.

It is especially useful as a place for socializing when more than one or two people are camping.

An outdoor shade shelter provides a large area with protection from sun and rain.

The open sides of a shade shelter make it especially appropriate for use as an outdoor cooking area.

The "footprint" is a piece of material made of the same fabric as the tent and that fits underneath it.

It provides protection from wear and tear and also is easier to clean than washing the whole tent.

Some mold avoiders report that the footprint is much less likely to grow mold than other ground covers, and so it may be worth the extra investment when buying a tent.

Tent Supplies

Especially when camping in the desert where the ground is hard, having a mallet or hammer to use to pound the tent stakes into the ground is absolutely essential.

Mallets are easy to lose, and so having an extra on hand may be a good idea.

Tent stakes come in a variety of different types.

The lighter, more expensive stakes tend to be best for backpacking.

Heavy steel stakes are more durable and functional for car camping.

The lack of tent stakes has the potential of ruining a wilderness camping experience if misplaced, and so carrying some extras is a good idea.

Sleeping

For most people pursuing mold avoidance for health reasons, the goal for a mattress is to find something that is tolerable in terms of off-gassing; that can be washed easily if it gets cross-contaminated; that will not be unpleasant on cold nights; and that will be relatively comfortable.

A usual choice is a self-inflating sleeping pad.

(Self-inflating is a bit of an exaggeration -- it may need a bit of help in blowing it up.)

These sleeping pads tend to be tolerated by people with a wide range of reactivities and are relatively comfortable even when the ground underneath is uneven or has rocks in it.

For people who are car camping, choosing a thick sleeping pad (such as 2" or even 3" thick) in the longest/widest size may be worth the small additional cost.

For those who would prefer not to sleep on the ground, a camping cot may be in order.

Pillows

Probably there is no item that is more important to have free of contamination than the pillow.

Even a slight amount of toxin on a pillow may shut down the body's detoxification activities during sleep and interfere with sound sleep.

Pillows need to be easily washable.

For instance, LL Bean has sold some washable camping pillows, in either flannel or down.

Another wholly washable option is to use a rolled-up towel as a pillow.

Since cotton takes a long time to dry, a microfiber camping towel might be considered for this.

Another possibility could be a small blanket or throw folded up and placed inside a pillowcase.

Some mold avoiders use no pillow at all - in which case, having the fabric underneath the head be free of toxins may be particularly important.

Whatever kind of "pillow" is used, having a few extras on hand is a good idea so that it can be switched for a different one if it starts to feel problematic partway through the night.

A "headboard" of some sort can make sleeping in a tent more comfortable, especially for people who want to read in bed.

A rolled-up blanket could serve this purpose, or a cloth laundry bag filled with spare clean clothes, or a wedge.

Sleeping Bags

Most of the sleeping bags that are found in stores like REI are the "mummy" type.

Mummy sleeping bags are good for trapping body heat for cold-weather sleeping and usually are fairly light (and therefore useful for backpacking).

The downside of mummy bags for people with pain or sleep issues is that they can be restrictive and uncomfortable.

Rectangular bags tend to be much roomier and more comfortable.

LL Bean makes a selection of rectangular bags (which also can be used as comforters) appropriate for different temperatures, for instance.

The main downside of rectangular bags is that they are relatively bulky and thus a bit of a challenge to wash by hand, meaning that avoiding cross-contamination is particularly important.

Down insulation in sleeping bags is more breathable but also conceivably might grow mold.

Synthetic insulation might be safer.

For cold-weather camping, using a mummy sleeping bag with a second rectangular bag unzipped as a comforter over the top can provide maximum warmth.

Regardless of what kind of sleeping bag is being used, a sleeping bag liner may be a good idea.

Unlined "mummy" bags tend to be slippery and uncomfortable, and having to wash larger bags by hand when they start to feel grungy is a lot of work.

Sleeping bag liners are available in a variety of materials, including fleece, silk, cotton and polyester.

For warm weather camping, sleeping bag liners can be used on their own without a bag.

Some mold avoiders suggest mylar sleeping bags, which are disposable and warm.

Of course, there is no reason why (especially in warm weather) anyone must use a sleeping bag at all.

If a bag feels too constricting or uncomfortable, then sticking with easily washable sheets and blankets may end up being a better choice.

Bedding

Cotton is not a very practical choice for camping blankets since it takes a long time to dry.

As a result, even those people who would never use anything other than cotton bedding back in civilization usually end up resorting to synthetic blankets when camping.

Certain wool blankets are designed to be washed occasionally and could be an option for people who are confident that they can keep cross-contamination at a minimum.

Note that wool tends to be a material that is hard to remediate from mold toxins, even when it is washed.

Regardless of whether sleeping bags are used, having several fleece blankets on hand may be a good idea.

Fleece blankets may be useful for extra warmth; as a pillow or bolster; to wrap around the sleeping pad to prevent slipping and sliding; or to spread on the ground for picnics.

Preferably blankets would be small (throw size might be best) for ease of washability.

Electric blankets may add a good bit of comfort to the camping experience when the weather is even a little cool, for those who can tolerate them and are camping with access to electricity.

Twin-sized sheets are a bit large for sleeping pads, but could be considered since they may be easier to hand wash than blankets.

Towels and Robes

Traditional cotton terrycloth towels take a very long time to dry and a large amount of room to store, and thus may not be very practical for camping.

Microfiber towels or waffle-weave cotton towels are alternatives that dry fast and take up less storage space.

Having at least one robe on hand is a good idea when camping (for instance, to wear after showering, swimming or spending time in hot springs).

A robe that dries fast, such as one made of waffle-weave cotton, may be most appropriate.

Bathing

If a shower is not available or is non-usable due to mold, here are some options for bathing outdoors.

The Zodi shower requires only batteries and a camping fuel canister to create a warm or hot 10-minute outdoor shower.

The Ecotemp shower hooks up directly to a garden hose, using propane fuel and batteries to create a warm showering experience.

The Nemo Helio Pressure Shower sits on the ground and uses a foot pump to create water pressure, with the sun heating up the water. (Water also could be heated up on a camp stove.) No batteries or propane tanks are required.

Traditional solar showers (often five gallon) heat up water in a solar-powered bag, providing a low-tech warm shower.

Though an inexpensive option, traditional solar showers have a number of disadvantages especially for people who are still ill.

The water in solar showers takes several hours to warm up (meaning that planning is required and multiple showers per day may not be feasible); a place to hang the bag overhead will be needed; and the individual needs to be strong enough to lift the fairly heavy bag to that high location.

Regardless of what other plans for washing are made, having a couple of large metal bowls on hand can be a good backup plan.

With warm water and mild soap in one basin, clear warm water in the second basin, and a wash cloth, a pretty effective sponge bath can be accomplished relatively quickly.

Bathing outdoors also requires consideration of modesty issues.

Although shower shelters are available, they generally take up a lot of space in the car, are difficult for one person to set up, and are not really appropriate for the propane-based showers.

For sponge baths, a tall tent would work for privacy.

Other options include showering in the open in a bathing suit or loose clothing, or showering in a secluded outdoor area.

Toilet

Almost all campgrounds and RV parks provide either conventional toilets or "pit toilets."

Mostly these are acceptable enough mold-wise to be usable, though there are some exceptions.

For those camping away from settled campgrounds, a small shovel will be needed to dig cat holes to bury stool.

Cooking

A wide variety of foods can be prepared on a camp stove, powered by propane gas in small tanks.

For car camping, the heavier models by Coleman are the most popular.

Coleman makes a stove with two burners; a model with a large grill; and a model with one burner and a smaller grill.

Although campers commonly use the grill on the latter model as a second burner, this is not something that Coleman recommends.

The grills on these Coleman stoves are made of aluminum.

For those concerned about aluminum toxicity, the use of a cast-iron grill pan (such as those made by Lodge) on a two-burner stove might be considered.

Coleman stoves work well on picnic tables.

For camping away from established campsites, a table of some sort to hold the grill stove and to eat on may be useful.

Although the small tanks of propane that power most camping stoves are available in many locations, they tend to be much more expensive out in the middle of nowhere than they are at, say, Wal-Mart.

Coleman's camping oven (designed to fit on the grill stove) is inexpensive, folds flat for storage and gets great reviews.

A solar oven is also a possibility.

With regard to cookware, flexibility is key in order to save space.

Most people find a frying pan and two saucepans (medium or large) to be a good starting point.

Especially for those who might consider cooking over an open fire, cast iron may be worth considering (though it takes some effort with regard to proper seasoning and maintenance).

Wal-Mart generally has a good selection of Lodge cast-iron pans.

A chopping board of some sort can be helpful.

Basic utensils used for cooking to consider bringing: chef's knife, paring knife, vegetable peeler, spatula, soup ladle, slotted spoon, solid spoon, tongs, can opener.

Some "specialty" tools (cheese grater, potato masher, citrus juicer) could be considered as well.

For coffee, some practical options include the Aeropress, a French press, a percolator, or a non-electric version of a drip coffee maker.

Refrigeration

Keeping food cool enough not to spoil is one of the bigger challenges in camping.

The simplest and least expensive option is to use a well-insulated cooler.

Provided that ice (available in close proximity to most campgrounds) is purchased frequently and the cooler is drained regularly, fresh or frozen food can last for an extended period of time in a regular cooler.

This does require a good bit of commitment with regard to maintaining the cooler on a regular basis.

A cooler with a spigot at the bottom to drain off water can be helpful for this.

Keeping food in some kind of smaller container inside the cooler so that it doesn't get wet may be worth considering.

A much more expensive alternative is a refrigerator powered by the cigarette lighter in the car or by a solar panel.

Engel and Norcold are popular brands.

These refrigerators may require less tending than a non-electric cooler and have the potential of keeping foods more solidly cold.

In hot weather, added ice may be necessary to keep food frozen in this type of refrigerator.

Dishes

The problem with using conventional dishes for camping is that they have the potential of breaking. They also tend to take up a lot of room in the car.

More practical choices of dishes for camping include enamelware (such as traditional blue camping style), Corelle or various plastic dishes.

Choosing plates (such as the traditional camping ones) that can serve as a holder for paper plates can save a lot of clean-up time.

Non-breakable coffee mugs can be made out of stainless steel or plastic.

Some kind of water glasses or water bottles will be needed.

Some people may prefer these to be glass even though it involves taking more care.

For hiking longer distances, multiple lightweight water bottles may be needed, since those with toxicity-related illnesses may not want to drink unfiltered water even if it is available on the trail.

Unless the goal is to save weight in backpacking, regular metal silverware is generally a fine choice.

A good insulated carafe to hold hot beverages can be very helpful when camping in cold weather, since having something hot to drink when waking up shivering in the middle of the night can make a big difference.

Some kind of improvised dish pan will be needed to wash dishes.

For instance, this could be a larger pot, one of the large bowls used for bathing, or a plastic storage bin used to store dishes or cookware when on the road.

Electronics

A challenge while camping is keeping electronic items charged.

Even when electricity is not available at the campsites, in many locations there is a spot in the vicinity where people can sit outdoors and charge their devices.

An inverter that plugs into the cigarette lighter of the car can be very useful in charging devices while on the road.

A solar panel could be used at the campsite.

Although many of the most pristine locations do not have cell phone service, often it is possible to find an Internet connection nearby.

Skype (possibly in voice-only mode) can be a good substitute for cell phone service, with calls to telephone numbers costing a modest fee.

An Amazon Kindle (possibly a basic one with a long battery life) can be a useful item, since books tend to get cross-contaminated easily and take up a lot of room in the car.

A portable DVD player - preferably with the longest battery life available - may be useful for watching movies in remote locations.

Other Electric Appliances

Most tent campers (especially those reliant on their laptops) end up with access to electricity at least some of the time.

Additional appliances using electricity therefore may be worth considering.

A slow cooker may be a good choice since it has the ability to make available a variety of foods that would be impractical or impossible to cook on a camp stove.

Juicers and high-speed blenders take up a good bit of room in the car and use a lot of electricity, though conceivably they may be worth bringing for people wanting to include more raw produce in their diets.

Much more practical for camping (with almost no cleanup) is an immersion blender, which can be used to puree cooked vegetables into soups or fruits into smoothies.

When camping in hot weather, an electric fan can be pleasant.

Furniture

A comfortable chair can make a big difference in terms of the enjoyment of a camping trip.

A camping stool takes up almost no room in the car and (especially when orthostatic intolerance is a problem) may be helpful on some occasions.

A small table that folds up flat (such as those sold by camping stores) may be useful in the tent or for the camp stove.

Light

Battery-operated headlamps provide hands-free light at night.

Having at least a couple of headlamps and plenty of batteries on hand is a good idea.

A bright battery-operated lantern can provide a safe general source of light, perhaps especially suited for use in the tent at night.

For more light for a longer period of time outdoors, consider a fuel-based lantern such as one that uses white gas.

Plenty of extra mantles are inexpensive and a good idea to have on hand when using a fuel-based lantern.

Heat

Desert or mountain areas can become cold at night, even when the temperatures are comfortable during the day.

Some mold avoiders have been helped when camping in cold weather by the use of electric or propane heaters to heat their tents.

This requires careful consideration of safety issues, however.

In addition, using the tent fly to hold in the heat can prevent desired air circulation.

Electric blankets can be very helpful, provided that individuals can tolerate them.

Another option for cold-weather camping are "instant heat" products, which can take the chill off cold hands or feet.

A hot water bottle is another possibility.

Water

In most campgrounds, water will be available at the campsite.

Having a container to carry water (maybe a collapsible one that won't take up much space) is a good idea in case it is not.

Since water quality can vary, it may be best to prepare for all possibilities -- for instance, to have on hand a water filter for use if the water is not irreparably contaminated plus some drinkable bottled water.

Laundry

With the recent emergence of particularly bad toxins associated with washing machines, using public laundry facilities is a risky endeavor for those pursuing mold avoidance.

Planning to do laundry by hand is a safer choice.

An in-depth discussion about laundry is in Chapter 38.

If a problem when camping is that there does not seem to be any place to hang a clothesline, consider asking for suggestions.

Some campgrounds (such as certain KOA's) forbid laundry from being hung outside.

This - along with anticipated water quality - is something to consider when planning where to do laundry on a road trip.

Often times, people who are camping intersperse their time in the wilderness with days spent in hotel rooms where clothing may be washed.

Having a collection of hangers on hand can be useful in hanging laundry to dry in the room during the hotel stay.

Clothes

It tends to be a good idea to have an ample supply of clean clothes on hand at all times, protected in plastic bins.

Extra clothing may come in handy if a problematic contamination occurs or if doing laundry becomes impractical for an extended period of time.

Even for people who have never worn fleece prior to doing avoidance, it can be a practical choice since it can be washed easily by hand and dries very fast.

Large coats (and especially ones that are not washable) tend to be not be a very good idea for mold avoiders.

Layers or down jackets tend to be much more practical.

Most people need to get out of their tent on occasion in the middle of the night, and nightgowns or pajamas tend not to be warm enough and also tend to lead to feelings of vulnerability.

Stretchy knit pants or sweatpants, loose knit tops and fleece jackets may be more appropriate for sleeping purposes.

If planning to camp in cold weather, proper accessories (hat, scarf, gloves, thick socks) will be appropriate at night as well as during the day.

Thinking about sleeping comfort when choosing these items may be a good idea.

Having shoes (such as clogs or flip-flops) available that can be easily removed and then put back on may be helpful for smoothly moving in and out of the tent.

Waterproof sandals to wear in public showers are a must.

Especially when sun is bright, good sunglasses are important. Sunlight has the potential of damaging the eyes (e.g. cataracts), perhaps especially in people with mold illness issues.

At least a couple of hats to provide protection from the sun as well as protection from getting hair cross-contaminated with mold are good thing to have on hand.

For hiking, good shoes or boots are important.

Good socks are probably even more important.

Even for most areas that qualify as desert, an umbrella and a rain jacket (possibly one that folds away compactly) can be useful.

Hiking

Especially for people whose coordination is not very good, a hiking staff or hiking poles can make hiking a much more enjoyable as well as safer activity.

Carrying an ample supply of water while hiking is very important.

A backpack or fanny pack likely will be needed to carry the water and other gear.

Other Items

A battery-operated tent ceiling fan can be helpful in increasing air circulation and providing a mild breeze in hot weather.

A supply of plastic garbage bags and paper towels on hand is a good idea for anyone pursuing mold avoidance, especially while camping.

Toilet paper and baby wipes may come in handy.

Considering that camping spots may be remote, carrying jumper cables in the car may be a good idea.

Especially when wash water is going to be dumped on the ground, all-natural biodegradable soap is preferable.

Dr. Bronner's liquid soap is a popular choice for bathing, doing dishes and washing clothes.

Some kind of small waterproof bag for toiletries is convenient.

Having several lighters (preferably the long ones) and a large supply of batteries on hand is a good idea.

For those who are not reactive to smoke, firewood and fire starters could be considered.

A first aid kit is always a good thing to have on hand.

Special tweezers to remove intact ticks may be considered.

For storage, plastic bins (available at Target or Wal-Mart) work well in terms of keeping things organized and protecting them from cross-contamination.

Plastic also can serve double duty as a basin for doing laundry or dishes.

Keeping all possessions in bins that can be easily removed from the car and stacked up if the need to sleep in the car occurs can provide more flexibility.

A tarp to cover the plastic bins and other belongings when they are stacked outside of the car may be worth considering.

Even with GPS, a good atlas can be helpful when traveling to unknown areas.

A compass for hiking (and for use in the car if GPS is not available) may be a good idea.

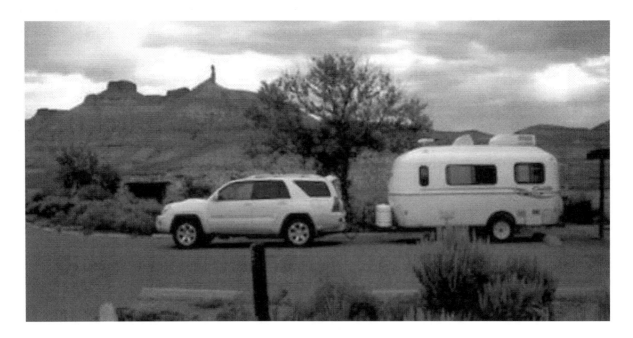

Flaming Gorge National Recreation Area near Green River, Wyoming.

Chapter 24

MECU

The Mobile Environmental Containment Unit (MECU) consists of an RV or other vehicle that is low in terms of problematic toxins.

It can be used as an adjunct to a conventional residence or as a full-time home.

For those pursuing mold avoidance, the MECU may have a number of benefits.

* It may allow people to spend more time in pristine locations in the wilderness while still enjoying some of the comforts of home.

* It may provide a safe place to decontaminate quickly while out and about.

* In areas where problematic outdoor toxins are only sporadically present, it may be moved from place to place in order to avoid toxic plumes.

* It may allow people to gain a sense of the extent to which toxins in the outdoors are having a negative effect on them, since the MECU will allow them to move from place to place without changing their indoor environment.

* It may provide a "Plan B" so that people are not left homeless if their main residence unexpectedly becomes too toxic to be safely inhabited by them.

Some downsides and difficulties of the MECU concept include the following.

* Most commercial RV's eventually acquire toxic mold problems.

* RV's that are likely to remain safe tend to be challenging to acquire or expensive.

* People who are starting out with avoidance and are still relatively sick may not have the energy or strength to handle an RV.

* Full-time RV living may soon start to feel confined or claustrophobic.

* Living full-time in an RV may not be appropriate for those with significant others or children.

* Some people respond negatively at an emotional level to the idea of living in or even occasionally sleeping in an RV.

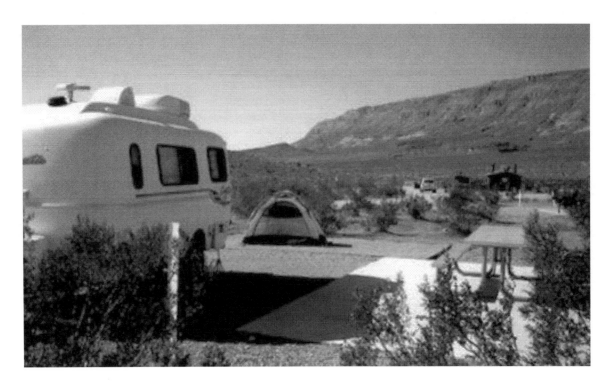

Red Rock Canyon National Conservation Area just outside Las Vegas, Nevada.

Chapter 25

Choosing the MECU

Although RV's have the potential of being beneficial for mold avoiders in a variety of ways, obtaining an RV that will not end up causing problems with regard to toxins can be a real challenge.

Most commercial RV's have hidden plywood in their construction.

Condensation almost always eventually causes mold growth that is impossible to remediate in these areas, making them inappropriate choices for those people pursuing mold avoidance.

In addition, almost all commercial RV's are made with materials that are quite toxic.

This means that they are likely to be a problem for anyone with even moderate chemical sensitivities for a considerable length of time after their manufacture.

The presence of chemicals also may be responsible for the observation that when mold is present in RV's, it tends to be particularly toxic mold.

Therefore, only a few types of RV's currently available seem really suitable for those pursuing mold avoidance.

Camplite

Camplite (made by Livin' Lite) is a fairly new RV brand that the company says is made mostly from aluminum and without any wood.

It is available as a travel trailer, a fifth wheel and a truck camper.

Like almost all commercial RV's, the Camplite uses chemicals that may make it intolerable to those who are reactive to manmade chemicals.

It may take many months of off-gassing - or even longer - for it to die down enough to be tolerated by most mold avoiders.

Thus far, relatively few used Camplites have become available on the marketplace.

Purchasing a new one and letting it sit for an extended period of time may be an option.

Possibly some dealers would sell demonstration models as well.

Although the Camplite includes styrofoam insulation, a downside of metal construction is that it tends to be especially cold in winter and hot in summer.

A positive factor is that metal tends to be relatively resistant to cross-contamination from mold toxins, including those in the outdoor air.

So far, Camplite trailers seem to hold their value well, making them a relatively safe choice for those concerned about protecting their financial assets.

Fiberglass RV's

A few mold avoiders have successfully lived in fiberglass RV's - such as Casita or Scamp - for extended periods of time.

Unlike most RV's, these fiberglass models do not have wood in the construction of the walls.

However, they do utilize wood (heavily coated with fiberglass) as the subfloor.

Although mold avoiders often seem to be able to tolerate this sort of RV, the wood in the floor eventually may be subject to mold growth.

These RV's seem to be somewhat more toxic with regard to manmade chemicals than the Camplite.

For some people, it may take years of off-gassing before they are tolerable.

A positive about these fiberglass trailers is that they are well-insulated and may be more comfortable in either hot or cold weather than metal RV's.

A downside is that fiberglass is easily cross-contaminated by outdoor toxins and may take a long time to recover from even transient exposures.

Fiberglass trailers that have spent time in particularly bad locations may not ever recover to the point of being usable by extreme reactors.

Casita is made in Texas.

Scamp is made in Minnesota.

Both Casita and Scamp make mid-sized trailers that can be towed with a truck or SUV, plus a small model (13') that can be towed with a regular car.

Scamp also makes a larger fifth wheel that can be towed only with a pickup truck.

Casita and Scamp tend to be extremely popular on the resale market and hold their value well.

Automobiles

Cars tend to be much less problematic in terms of mold growth than RV's.

Although cars can become moldy too, the lack of wood in their construction is a plus with regard to this problem.

New cars generally are less of a problem than new RV's with regard to chemicals as well.

The main mold issue in cars tends to be associated with the air conditioning system.

Many mold avoiders purchase cars without air conditioning or even have the air conditioning system removed.

Not running the air conditioning may not be sufficient since in some vehicles, running just the heat can lead to mold growth in the air conditioning system.

Especially for mold avoiders who are not planning to have access to an RV, choosing a vehicle that can be slept in comfortably may be a good idea.

This will make it easier to get out to areas with good air and will serve as a "Plan B" if something happens to the primary residence.

A few options that might allow comfortable sleeping include a van, an SUV, a pickup truck with shell on top, or a Honda Element or Toyota Matrix (both now out of production but often available used).

Many healthy people have made modifications to their vans in order to be able to live out of them in reasonable comfort, and a great deal of information is available on this topic.

For extended trips or for those choosing to live a camping lifestyle out of the car, towing a small utility trailer could be an option.

Belongings could be stored in the trailer, or a bed could be kept in it.

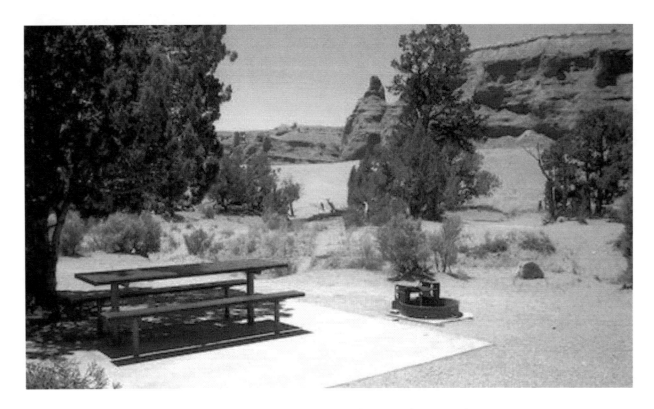

Kodachrome Basin State Park in southern Utah.

Chapter 26

MECU Conversion

The main reason to consider converting a utility trailer into a livable home is to avoid the issues with toxicity inherent in commercial RV's.

Utility trailers generally do not use buried wood in their construction and thus will not have the hidden mold problems that so often plague commercial RV's.

They also generally do not use the glues and other toxic chemicals that are so often substantial problems in new commercial RV's.

In addition, a conversion of this type can include only the features that are needed rather than the RV manufacturer's standard features.

A utility trailer conversion can be put together with modular components, making it easier to remove the offending item if contamination occurs.

Depending on the choices that are made, a utility trailer conversion can be significantly less expensive than a commercial RV.

The main downside of a conversion is finding someone to do the work at an acceptable price (or, for those who are handy, doing the work yourself).

An additional possible downside is that the finished product might not be as aesthetically attractive as a commercial RV.

A Simple Box

The utility trailer on its own has the potential of being an inexpensive, bare-bones refuge that is still more comfortable than sleeping in an automobile or tent.

Depending on the size, it may cost $2,000 to $4,000.

Choosing a unit with adequate ventilation (such as a window and a rooftop vent) may be important for mold avoiders, since a primary purpose of obtaining an MECU is to get more exposure to good-quality air.

A long extension cord could serve to bring electricity into the trailer.

An electric hot plate could be used for indoor cooking or heating water, or a gas stove could be used outdoors.

Wash basins could be used for sponge baths indoors.

While many people would not want to live in this sort primitive domicile for an extended period of time, some people may find it much preferable to other options that they might have available at a particular point in their lives.

Getting Conversions Done

Most cargo trailer manufacturers have the ability to add on a wide variety of options at the factory for a relatively low price.

Some options available may include electricity, batteries, side door, roof-top vent, dome light, foam insulation and electric brakes.

Considering the cost of hiring someone to add these options, it may be worthwhile to order a cargo trailer new to get them installed rather than buying a used one.

Additional conversion options may require finding someone to install them, which tends to run a premium with regard to labor costs.

Following is a discussion of some basic features that may be added to a plain utility trailer to make it more livable.

Electricity

Electric wiring may make the trailer feel much more livable than just using an extension cord.

Batteries of the type used in RV's can be useful for having small amounts of electricity available when camping away from power sources.

A solar panel could be added to the roof of the RV.

While solar panels do not generate large amounts of power (and only work on sunny days), they may be helpful for supplying light, keeping electronics devices charged, running a water pump, and running other appliances that take only a small amount of electricity.

Electric generators convert gasoline into electricity.

Though noisy, they provide a reliable source of electricity anywhere.

Connecting the electricity to the truck or other tow vehicle will charge the batteries and keep the refrigerator working while on the road.

Thinking carefully about where to place electric lights and plugs in the RV may make it feel more livable.

Insulation

Especially when camping in very cold places or very hot places, insulation is an important consideration.

Styrofoam is often used as insulation by those pursuing mold avoidance.

Some styrofoam is better in terms of VOC's than others, so it may be best to check samples out in person before committing.

Some people in cold climates put substantial amounts of styrofoam (such as 6") on the floor as well as on the ceiling and walls.

Hiding the styrofoam behind a wall covering may be desirable for aesthetics.

Metal sheeting may be preferred to cover the styrofoam, since plastic tends to absorb mycotoxins particularly well.

During the summer months, a reflective piece of aluminum on the roof of the trailer or a shade shelter may be helpful in keeping things cooler.

Plumbing

Installing plumbing in a trailer is a fairly challenging endeavor that will add to the cost substantially if done professionally.

Therefore, the first question that needs to be determined is whether this is actually necessary or desirable.

A discussion of this topic is in Chapter 27.

Ventilation

For good air circulation, one or more windows plus a rooftop vent fan may be desirable.

Multiple windows may allow more ventilation and also give a more attractive feeling to the trailer.

However, windows also may draw more attention to the trailer when it is parked overnight in areas where camping is not allowed (such as on city streets).

Windows also are an added expense.

Window coverings of some kind likely will be needed.

For ease of entry and exit, a side door (in addition to the back loading doors already on the trailer) may be useful.

Heating and Cooling

Air conditioners very often tend to become moldy.

Many mold avoiders use no air conditioning at all (and think of sweating as detoxifying and thus a good thing).

For those who have temperature regulation problems, a small portable air conditioner that can be disposed of if it becomes moldy may be preferable to one that is attached more permanently to the vehicle.

When camping with electricity, one or two portable electric heaters generally will be enough to heat a medium-sized insulated RV to a comfortable temperature, even when it is below freezing outside and even when windows are open for ventilation.

For those who can tolerate them, an electric blanket may be helpful.

For camping in winter in places without electricity, a propane heater (portable or installed) could be considered.

Propane heaters may trigger chemical sensitivities and have safety issues, however.

A small wood stove is also a possibility.

Kitchen

RV refrigerators are meant to run on propane gas, electricity or battery power.

They may have buried cardboard in them with the potential of going moldy.

They also are relatively expensive.

A portable refrigerator/freezer that runs on both AC and DC current may be an option for those who plan to camp primarily in places with electricity (and to use power from the car to keep the refrigerator going while on the road).

An inexpensive electric refrigerator (with a cooler using ice as backup) may be sufficient for those who plan to camp mostly in places with electricity.

This kind of refrigerator will not be working when driving, however.

Ventilating the refrigerator properly to avoid the accumulation of exhaust gases is important.

For cooking, a portable propane stove (for outdoor use) or an electric hotplate could be used.

Some more expensive propane stoves are advertised as being appropriate for indoor use as well.

A slow cooker, toaster oven or small microwave also could be considered.

Furniture

Camping cots can be very comfortable and are an obvious choice for a bed.

A bench that would hold a mattress also could be built into the conversion.

Some kind of table and chair for eating and working may be considered.

A comfortable chair of some sort may be desirable.

Keeping Things Secure

A main challenge in RV living is keeping things secure so that they don't move around and possibly break while on the road.

This means that cabinets or closets that are firmly attached to the walls may be especially important to keep items contained.

Considering how to store items such as furniture so that they do not move around while on the road is important as well.

A bungee cord system is often useful.

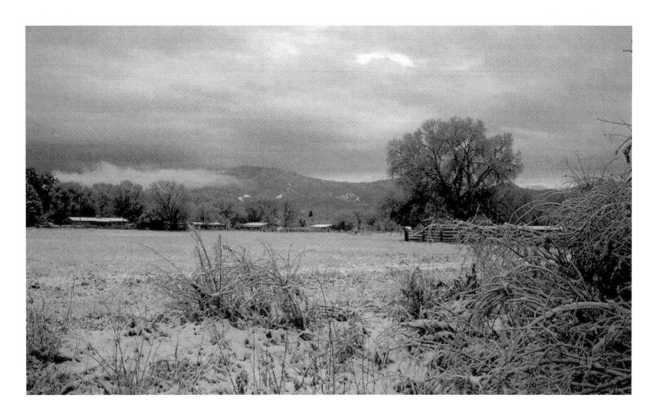

Taos, New Mexico.

Chapter 27

MECU Plumbing

Having plumbing in the MECU has good points and bad points for those pursuing mold avoidance.

On the upside, plumbing makes decontamination much easier - meaning that mold avoiders are more likely to do it as often as necessary.

It also can make RV living feel more civilized and thus more tolerable from an emotional standpoint for long-term living.

However, plumbing also has the potential of leading to toxic mold growth in the holding tanks or drainpipes of the RV.

In addition, a hidden leak may result in mold growth.

Since neither using plumbing nor not using plumbing is ideal, mold avoiders need to decide whether to have it based on their own personal circumstances and priorities.

Conventional RV Plumbing

Conventional RV plumbing is designed to create an experience that is as much like using the plumbing at home as possible.

Three tanks are installed under the RV: freshwater (filled with tap water), gray water (water already used for washing), and black water (sewage).

Black water and gray water are periodically removed from the RV at dump stations.

For people staying at RV parks, the gray water is usually continually drained through a hose into the sewer hookup, with black water periodically dumped.

Exhaust pipes from the black water and gray water tanks remove gasses and some of the odor from the RV tanks, usually through the roof.

A water pump (running on electricity or battery power) propels the freshwater to the sinks, shower and toilet.

Smaller RV's generally have a small bathroom (with shower, sink and toilet all in one space) as well as running water at the kitchen sink.

An advantage of this is that it creates a comfortable kitchen and bathroom experience.

It also gives mold avoiders a private place to do coffee enemas, a treatment that many individuals say has been helpful to them.

However, plumbing does introduce an element of risk to the enterprise.

Insofar as the RV does not contain any wood, the possibility that there might be a pipe leak is somewhat less worrisome.

The possibility that toxic mold may grow in black water and gray water tanks still may be a concern, however.

Because the most problematic microbial toxins become worse when treated with chemicals, avoiding conventional "anti-mold" products in holding tanks may be a good idea.

Some mold avoiders have found homemade milk kefir - which contains beneficial bacteria that may eliminate any mold spores that might be introduced into the tanks as well as reduce odors – to be a better choice.

The more that an RV is exposed to locations that have problematic mold toxins, the more preferable it may be to avoid a conventional tank system since the problematic spores may have the potential of settling into the tanks and growing.

Dumping waste into sewer systems that have been observed to be contaminated with particularly problematic mold toxins probably should be avoided as well, since spores may make their way up the sewer hose into the tanks.

No Plumbing

Some mold avoiders decide that plumbing is not necessary for them in their MECU.

Therefore, if they are putting together their own RV's, they do not install it.

In some cases, people living in RV's that already contain plumbing systems make the decision not to use those systems.

Many of these individuals plan on staying in places such as RV parks where bathroom facilities are available.

Such places often have outdoor sinks where dishes can be washed as well.

Planning to rely on public bathrooms is based on the hope that these bathroom facilities are not going to be too moldy to use.

Experiences suggest that while campground or RV park bathrooms with showers often do have some moderately toxic mold, it often is possible for even quite reactive people to use them.

Rinsing hair outside after the shower to remove cross-contamination may help to decrease the effects of a problematic shower area.

If public showers are not available, then not having tanks in the RV often means showering outdoors (see Chapter 23 on camping gear for options).

A sponge bath using water basins could be set up inside the RV for privacy.

Other than inconvenience, the main drawback of not having plumbing in an MECU is that it can make getting clear through proper decontamination on a regular basis much more difficult to achieve.

Alternative Plumbing

Frustrations with RV plumbing have led some mold avoiders to develop alternative systems.

One approach is to eliminate the black water tank but keep gray water, thus eliminating the need to take the risk of hooking up to sewer systems.

Since gray water is just wash water, it can be collected in a bucket and disposed of by pouring it down a drain or (in many places) dumped on the ground.

If the gray water tank is also a concern, then conceivably that tank could be eliminated even if wash water in the RV is still used.

Gray water could drain from the RV into a bucket underneath, which then could be tossed.

Some kind of pulley system likely would make this easier.

If desired, a composting toilet or other portable toilet could be added for those occasions when a public toilet is not available or is too toxic to use.

Those with experience in using portable toilets in their RV's suggest that the easiest method is to collect only urine (which then can be dumped easily into a sink) in the portable toilet.

Stool is more easily collected in a plastic bag filled with unscented kitty litter, sawdust or other composting material and then thrown away, they report.

Part 4

SUPER TOXINS

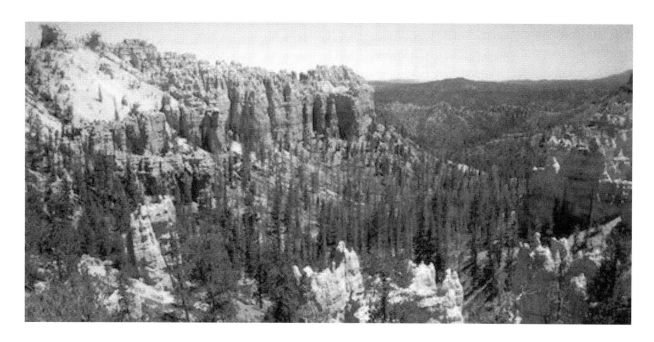

Bryce Canyon National Park in southern Utah.

Chapter 28

Super Toxin Overview

Although many different kinds of molds manufacture toxins, only a very small percentage of the time do molds make toxins that are catastrophically problematic for those who are hyperreactive to mold toxins.

Learning to accurately identify these super toxins and to take special care in avoiding them can allow mold avoiders to manage their health symptoms much more effectively than if they were trying to avoid all toxins in the same ways.

In addition, learning to recognize problem toxins can make mold avoiders' lives easier, since they then will be able to be less extreme in avoiding less dangerous toxins than they are in avoiding more dangerous toxins.

This following chapters in this section include some observations about some commonly encountered super toxins.

Reports suggest that all of these toxins have a universally problematic effect on individuals who are exposed to them (and to some healthy individuals as well).

The names are the ones commonly used by mold avoiders to refer to these toxins.

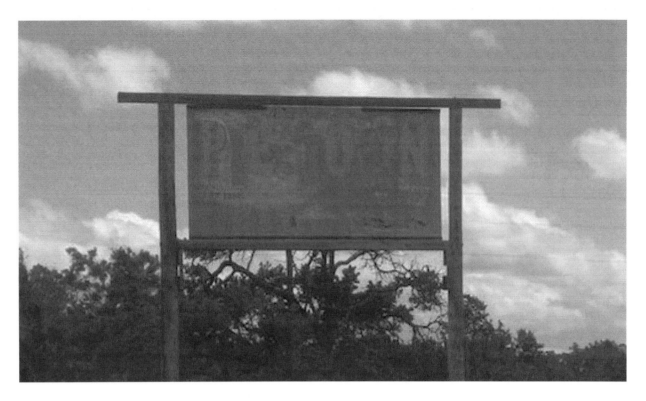

Pie Town, a tiny town at 7000 feet on the Continental Divide in western New Mexico.

Chapter 29

Super Stachy

Stachybotrys chartarum is a common indoor mold.

It is capable of growing on cellulose when even a small amount of standing water is present.

The large amounts of cellulose (including drywall, wall insulation, and dust in HVAC systems) in modern indoor environments have provided a fertile environment for Stachybotrys growth.

Many buildings contain at least small amounts of Stachybotrys.

A high percentage of buildings (such as 20% in many locations) contain enough Stachy to present problems for those pursuing mold avoidance.

Stachybotrys is capable of making a variety of trichothecenes as well as other toxins.

Trichothecenes have been shown in thousands of peer-reviewed papers to produce negative effects on almost every system of the body.

The most studied effects involve systems of the body that tend to be particularly problematic in chronic multisystem disease: the neurological system, the immune system and the intestinal system.

Anecdotally, ordinary Stachybotrys toxin seems to be moderately problematic in small quantities for mold avoiders.

Exposures to larger quantities (such as to buildings contaminated with a great deal of it) can prompt a variety of symptoms related to inflammation.

Occasionally in buildings contaminated with Stachybotrys, a much stronger version of a similar toxin will be present.

This toxin has the potential of cross-contaminating to a relatively high extent and of prompting symptoms in very tiny amounts.

This stronger version seems to be a fairly rare toxin, currently present in perhaps 1-2% of US buildings.

Anecdotally, many individuals with chronic multisystem disease first get sick or decline substantially when living in buildings with substantial amounts of this super toxin.

The exact nature of this toxin is unclear.

It could be that only certain strains of Stachy make this particularly problematic toxin.

It could be that another microorganism often grows in conjunction with Stachy and makes the problem toxin.

Or it could be that this super toxin is actually a combination of toxins, interacting synergistically to be particularly harmful.

Another possibility is that regular Stachybotrys manufactures much more harmful toxins when it comes into contact with certain environmental chemicals.

The use of flea bombs is particularly suspected as having the potential to convert Stachybotrys from an ordinarily problematic toxin producer into an extremely problematic one.

The super toxin associated with Stachybotrys has the potential of permanently cross-contaminating items that have been exposed to it for extended periods of time.

Usually this toxin can be washed off after short exposures.

This toxin seems to produce a high amount of oxidative stress, with the bodies of those being affected compensating by reducing the amount of oxygen being used throughout the system.

This tends to result in extreme physical and mental sluggishness, amongst other symptoms.

The tendency of many affected individuals to be lethargic with regard to either cleaning up the mold or leaving a bad environment may be related to this.

Regular Stachy is also known to have a negative effect on the immune system and to cause brain damage (including the creation of perforations in the blood-brain barrier).

Trichothecenes in general are known to cause leaky gut and other issues related to the small intestine.

Particularly severe manifestations of these health problems tend to be associated with exposures to the super toxin version of Stachy.

Mold avoiders also tend to experience negative emotional changes and cognitive effects (such as brain fog and disruption of executive function) upon being exposed to even small amounts of this super toxin.

Larger amounts have the potential of prompting more dramatic negative effects in those who are already clear - for instance, the feeling of being hit on the back of the head with a frying pan.

Usually a quick decontamination is very helpful in reducing the effects of this super toxin.

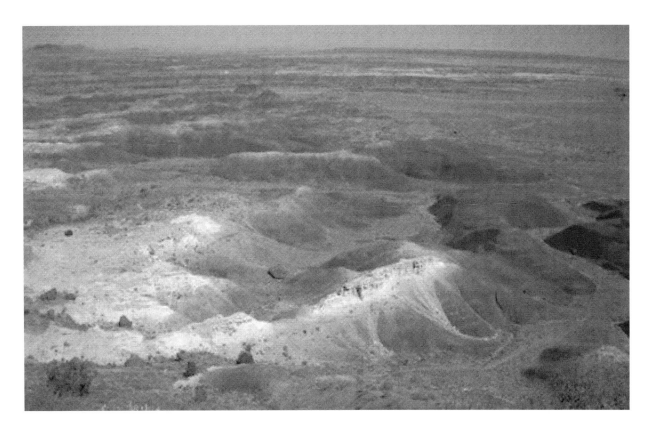

The Painted Desert in northeastern Arizona.

Chapter 30

Mystery Toxin

A quite different toxin is variously known as the "Tahoe Toxin," the "Berkeley Toxin," the "Mystery Toxin" and "Ick" (an abbreviation for idiopathic contaminant or "IC").

This toxin is mostly found outdoors.

Usually it emanates from sewers, sewer ponds, compost farms or similar places where standing water meets human-made debris for extended periods of time.

The toxin affects mold-reactive people in profound ways, but it has some curious characteristics that prevent most people from knowing that they are being exposed to it.

This is the basis for the suggestion that it is a "mystery" toxin.

Immediate symptoms prompted by the Mystery Toxin tend to be relatively mild.

Usually mood changes (particularly a profound sort of depression or out-of-control anger), a stabbing feeling in the heart or sternum, or heart palpitations are the only giveaways.

More problematic symptoms generally do not set in until 4-36 hours after the initial exposure.

Since the Mystery Toxin has the potential of prompting very severe symptoms in sufferers, learning to identify warning signs and then taking appropriate action when exposed can be very important.

Usually, this toxin emerges outdoors during times when the barometric pressure is falling rapidly.

It is more common in the northern hemisphere from November through February (and seems to be largely responsible for why many individuals with chronic multisystem disease decline during the winter months).

Very occasionally, this toxin is present inside buildings.

Reports suggest that it may be more likely to present in buildings where there has been a sewer backup, standing water in a crawl space, or some other encroachment from the outdoors.

Individuals living in these buildings often become very ill.

Exposure to outdoor Mystery Toxin seems to have the ability to make healthy people feel temporarily uncomfortable or unhappy.

However, only in a few observed cases has it alone been sufficient to drive individuals into chronic multisystem illness, without exposure to particularly problematic buildings also being a factor.

Most cities have at least a small amount of this toxin in the air, emerging especially during the winter months.

A few locations (mostly cities) have a much larger problem with this toxin and are not good places for mold avoiders to live.

Very occasionally, this toxin is present in smaller towns or rural areas as well.

The toxin remains airborne on the wind for a substantial length of time, often blowing long distances (such as hundreds of miles) on plumes.

In some cases, entire cities or regions can be affected.

In others, smaller plumes may make some parts of a town very problematic while others remain mostly clear of it.

The propensity of this toxin to cross-contaminate is quite high.

Possessions that are cross-contaminated with this toxin can feel much worse during downturns in barometric pressure (due to weather shifts or being brought to a high altitude), even in places where the outdoor air is clear.

Cars that have spent time in areas with a great deal of this toxin may be impossible to remediate.

In many cases, items that are transiently contaminated with this toxin can be remediated by rinsing with water.

However, in other cases, even short exposures to this toxin can cause items to be impossible to remediate to the tolerance of severe reactors.

Symptoms resulting from Mystery Toxin tend to be quite distinct.

They are more similar to symptoms reported in the literature about aquatic biotoxins than they are to the symptoms reported with regard to most molds.

Warning Symptoms

Symptoms often experienced immediately upon exposure include the following.

* Heart pain (in particular, a feeling of a needle through the heart).

* Chest pressure (a feeling of a dagger through the chest or a marble – sometimes actually swollen – at the sternum).

* Heart palpitations.

* Loss of sense of direction (e.g. driving around randomly).

* Seizures or "white-outs" (where the brain goes 100% blank for extended periods of time, sometimes even when a concerted effort is being made to bring up thoughts).

* Stuck thinking (e.g. spend all day clicking on the same three websites or playing mindless Facebook games).

* Strong feelings of empty, hopeless depression (unrelated to circumstances).

* Feeling of skin being mildly burned.

* Feeling of sore throat.

Delayed Symptoms

Symptoms that often are delayed for a relatively short period of time (such as a few hours) can include the following.

* Extreme photophobia (light sensitivity).

* Extreme noise sensitivity.

* Cognitive problems that go beyond brain fog (e.g. inability to add numbers or recognize words).

* Weird memory losses (e.g. inability to remember the name of one's hometown or to find the way home).

* Severe trembling.

* Paralysis (literal paralysis or feelings of paralysis; often one-sided).

* Strong suicidal feelings.

* Feelings of paranoia, like people who are usually friends have become enemies.

* Strong feelings of anger and lack of inhibition in expressing it.

* Other emotions that are bizarrely inappropriate to the situation.

* Convulsions.

* Extreme MCS.

* Marked gait problems.

* Inability to sit or stand up (including severe POTS).

* Extremely deep skin "dents."

* Veins pop out of skin (look "ropy").

* Reactivation of herpes viruses (and emergence of related illnesses such as shingles, Bell's palsy or herpes simplex lesions).

After Effects

Symptoms that tend to be delayed for a longer period of time (such as a day or more) include the following:

* Excruciating headaches (migraine-like but not one-sided).

* Organ pain (particularly kidney pain).

* Fibromyalgia pain.

* Feeling of "fire ants walking through bone marrow."

More Information

Additional information about this toxin (including a list of locations where it often has been observed to be present) can be found in the Paradigm Change blog post, "Outdoor Toxins of Particular Relevance to Mold Illness Patients."

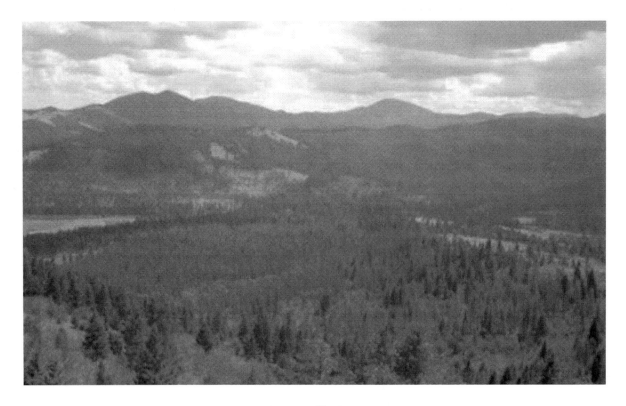

Near Great Falls, Montana.

Chapter 31

Hell Toxin

"Hell Toxin" is a particularly problematic substance that has been reported by increasing numbers of mold avoiders since 2013.

It also has been called the "Uber Toxin," the "Itch Toxin" and the "Hell Fire Toxin."

Reports about the Hell Toxin are very consistent across mold avoiders.

The most obvious effects of the toxin are strong feelings of skin burning (thus accounting for the name) that increase over time with ongoing exposure.

In some cases, very severe burns (similar to those seen in Stevens-Johnson syndrome) have been experienced.

In smaller amounts, this toxin may cause feelings of itchiness or prickliness rather than burning.

Rashes may also occur.

Negative emotional effects (such as severe depression or suicidal feelings) also tend to be associated with this toxin.

Although the dermatological and emotional symptoms tend to be the most identifiable effects of this toxin, it has been reported to have a very deleterious overall effect on the health of those exposed to it.

In addition, this toxin has the ability to cross-contaminate to what seems a ridiculous extent, even compared to other toxins.

In most cases, very mild burning and a feeling of emotional fear are the only presenting symptoms when people first come into contact with this toxin.

Therefore, acting proactively in order to avoid it may be worthwhile.

Here are some thoughts about doing that.

* The toxin is present to an increasingly large extent in many public buildings. In particular, certain laptop computers have been reported to be badly contaminated with the toxin and to be spreading it to places such as cafes and libraries. Avoiding places where laptops are frequently used or being especially careful about decontaminating after visiting these places may be a good idea.

* This toxin has repeatedly been reported to "explode" (possibly grow) in automatic washing machines. Therefore, hand washing all clothing that has been worn to public places may be advisable. Use of public laundry machines should be considered to be a particular risky endeavor.

* Once an item is contaminated with Hell Toxin, it very often is impossible to remediate it. If an item becomes contaminated with something that causes severe burning or itching, it may be best to consider the idea of just throwing the item out since this may make cross-contamination less likely.

* A few reports suggest that Hell Toxin has the potential of growing in sewers and cross-contaminating shoes. It thus may be best (especially in cities) to treat shoes as potentially cross-contaminated with this toxin and to deal with them appropriately (such as storing them in a box outside the living space so that they are less likely to cross-contaminate it).

* The emergence of this toxin makes maintaining a safe space particularly important. Being very cautious about decontaminating scrupulously before or immediately upon

entering the safe space as well as about introducing new items into the safe space may be a good idea.

More Information

This toxin is discussed in the section called "A Toxin that Itches and Burns" in the Paradigm Change blog post called "Outdoor Toxins of Particular Relevance to Mold Illness Patients."

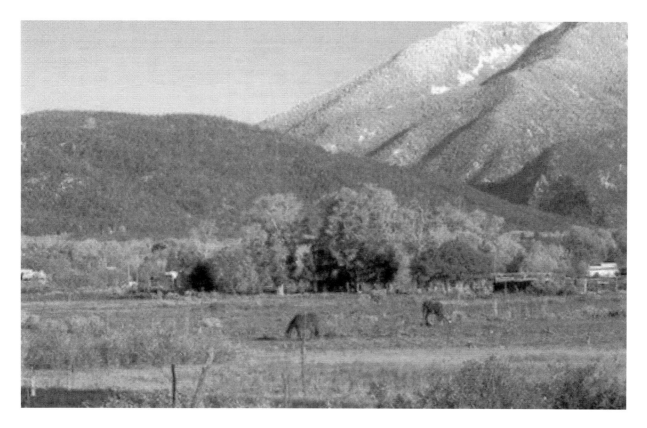

Arroyo Seco, New Mexico.

Chapter 32

Stealth Toxin

This super toxin has been less frequently reported than others discussed here.

However, when this toxin has been noted, it usually has been in the homes of individuals ill with chronic multisystem disease.

Reports suggest that this toxin tends to not be immediately noticeable at first, even to experienced mold avoiders who have encountered it before.

Cognitive issues eventually emerge, with other symptoms following later on.

This toxin seems to cross-contaminate to a substantial extent (though not nearly as much as has been reported about Hell Toxin).

Being constantly aware of one's cognitive abilities and departing quickly from environments that seem to be causing cognitive abilities to decline is one strategy for dealing with this toxin.

Part 5

AVOIDANCE TACTICS

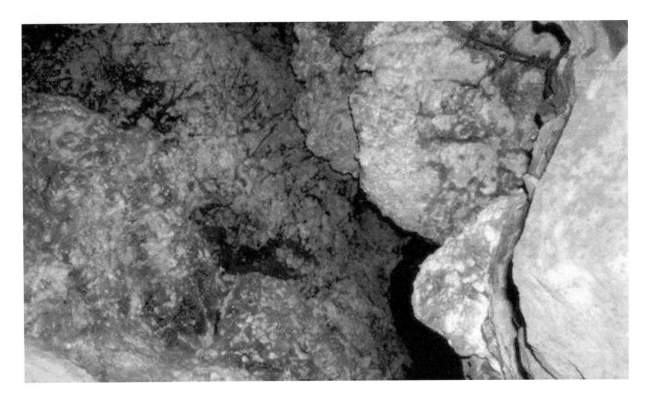

Jewel Cave National Park in the Black Hills of South Dakota.

Chapter 33

Detecting Mold

Those who succeed at making improvements through mold avoidance generally become very good at detecting whether problematic mold toxins are present in an environment or on an object based on their own reactions.

The goal here is to be able to immediately identify when particular toxins are present and, based on anticipated reactions, take appropriate steps to avoid them.

For some toxins, this may require minimal avoidance (such as taking a shower later in the day after returning home).

For other toxins, much more aggressive action (such as immediately decontaminating) may be deemed necessary.

It takes some practice to determine the warning symptoms associated with particularly problematic toxins, so that appropriate actions can be taken to avoid them.

Once this skill is obtained, mold avoidance may become less difficult and less frustrating.

Although reactions vary substantially depending on the toxin, and although different people sometimes have different reactions to the same toxin, here are some typical reactions.

Sight and Smell

Smell is not a very good indicator of the presence of particularly bad mold toxins.

Many buildings that are very problematic do not smell at all like mold, and some buildings that smell musty do not contain any toxic mold (or contain only mildly toxic mold).

The most problematic mold toxins do not have any smell at all, in the quantities required to cause substantial harm to mold avoiders.

Water marks on ceiling tiles generally are good indications that Stachybotrys or other cellulose-consuming molds are present and thus that the building will be problematic.

Stachybotrys usually grows hidden inside walls.

When Stachy can be seen, it usually looks more like smears of dirt on the wall than mold.

Other mold growth in buildings may be toxic or non-toxic.

Mold growing on food is usually non-toxic or only mildly toxic, but there are exceptions.

Outdoor mold is usually non-toxic or mildly toxic, but there are exceptions to that too.

Neurological

A variety of mold toxins have the ability to affect brain function.

Often this can result in symptoms such as forgetting words, losing track of the conversation, or periods where the mind goes completely blank.

Getting hopelessly lost can be a symptom of exposure to certain toxins, especially Mystery Toxin.

Executive functioning deficits (such as inability to organize or plan) can be indicative of exposures to mold toxins.

Brain fog seems to stem from general inflammation, very often triggered by mold exposures.

Convulsions where the body twitches involuntarily (sometimes severely) can be associated either with the aftermath of exposures or with detox.

Feelings of paralysis are experienced by some individuals subsequent to being hit with the Mystery Toxin or other toxins.

In some cases, actual paralysis where normal movement is not possible may be experienced.

Altered gait seems possibly related to the paralysis issue and also may manifest subsequent to an exposure.

Emotional

Unusual emotional symptoms that are way out of proportion to the situation being experienced are often indicative of exposures to mold toxins.

Emotional shifts often are the only immediate indication of exposure.

They thus should be monitored carefully and taken seriously.

Suicidal ideation (especially when the thoughts arise spontaneously for little or no reason) very often tends to be indicative of exposures to particularly problematic super toxins.

Feelings that friends have suddenly become enemies are often indicative of exposure to certain environmental toxins, especially Mystery Toxin.

Feelings of anger, loss of self-confidence, panic, anxiety, depression or other emotions that are overblown compared to the current situation (but nonetheless may seem to the person entirely justified) are very typical of exposures to certain mold toxins.

The Paradigm Change blog post called "The Depression Response" discusses the use of emotional responses to gauge environmental exposures.

Sleep

Sleep quality in a good environment tends to differ substantially from sleep quality in a problematic environment.

In a problematic environment, sleep tends to be impaired.

Individuals spending the night in bad environments tend to have difficulty falling asleep, often remain in a twilight state of partial sleep rather than moving into deep sleep, and almost always wake up feeling unrefreshed.

Drugs such as Klonopin or other benzodiazapines often are used to try to counter these sleep problems.

In a good environment, sleep tends to be much deeper.

Individuals may sleep for longer periods of time and feel like they are almost comatose during sleep.

The tendency of the body to go into deep sleep mode when in a good place may be an indication that it is working to detoxify exposures that were acquired previously.

Since sleeping deeply for extended periods of time can be very productive, this may be considered a positive symptom of healing rather than a problem.

Heart

Certain toxins (especially the Mystery Toxin) tend to be associated with symptoms associated with the heart.

This can often manifest as the feeling of a stabbing sensation in the heart or sternum.

The stabbing can feel like it is being made by anything from a sewing needle to a dagger.

A related sensation may be a feeling of swelling (sometimes actually swollen like a small marble) in the sternum.

Heart palpitations or rapid heartbeat often are indicators of exposure to especially problematic toxins as well.

Often heart symptoms occur immediately upon exposure.

Heart symptoms tend to be indicative of particularly bad toxins that should be avoided scrupulously, even if the warning symptoms feel mild.

Autonomic

Certain toxins (especially the Mystery Toxin) have the ability to prompt feelings of being chilled, including actual shivering.

Even when they are not associated with feeling cold, tremors can be a direct result of exposure to certain kinds of mold toxins.

Feeling suddenly hungry or having sudden sugar cravings can be a symptom of being hit with mold toxin.

Increased intolerance to noise, light or other stimuli can be an exposure symptom.

Chemical sensitivities often increase dramatically after exposure to the Mystery Toxin (and perhaps also to other mold toxins).

Usually these kinds of symptoms emerge a few hours after being hit.

Respiratory

Often sensitized people being exposed to a variety of different mold toxins will find it difficult to draw a deep breath.

This tends to be an immediate exposure symptom.

Skin

Hell Toxin is primarily identified by strong burning or itching sensations.

In some cases, actual burns that are very severe may occur from Hell Toxin exposures.

Hives or rashes also may be a symptom of this toxin.

Other mold toxins can create milder feelings of burning or itching.

Itching and burning sensations tend to be immediately noticeable with exposures and (for the most part) to go away with decontamination.

Often they increase in intolerability over time, as individuals are repeatedly exposed to the problem toxins.

Some people have reported that skin symptoms did not emerge for a day or two after they were first exposed to Hell Toxin but that the symptoms later became very severe.

Orthostatic Intolerance

Symptoms related to orthostatic intolerance (including postural orthostatic tachycardia or POTS) very often manifest following exposure to the Mystery Toxin.

Other toxins also may have the ability to lead to these symptoms.

Usually these symptoms manifest within a day or so after being exposed.

Pain

Both fibromyalgia pain and severe headaches (similar to migraines but not one-sided) tend to be likely to manifest as a delayed symptom after exposure to particularly problematic toxins (including the Mystery Toxin).

Fibromyalgia also may be associated with detoxification of stored toxins, including detox occurring as a result of being in a very clear place.

In more severely affected patients, pain may occur in organs associated with detoxification (such as liver, kidneys or spleen) subsequent to an exposure.

A few mold avoiders have noted a sensation that feels like "fire ants walking through the bone marrow" subsequent to exposures to the Mystery Toxin.

Insofar as these symptoms occur as a result of an exposure, the delay is usually a day or two.

Feelings of Being Poisoned

Stomach discomfort and vomiting can occur subsequent to exposures to some toxins as well as during detoxification.

The vomit has the potential of feeling quite acrid.

In some cases, blood (such as from menstruation or from a bloody nose) may feel very toxic subsequent to an exposure.

Toxic urine or stool may cause burning or have an unusual odor.

Insofar as these symptoms are due to a current exposure rather than the release of toxins previously stored in tissues, they tend to emerge within a day or two.

Pathogens

Many mold toxins have a direct impact on the immune system.

Emergence of pathogens may result subsequent to exposures to these toxins.

Candida flares (evidenced by a white coating on the tongue) are frequent.

Herpes viruses of all types often become more problematic after exposures to certain toxins (especially the Mystery Toxin), with herpes simplex or shingles outbreaks commonly seen.

Symptoms tend to show up within a couple of days of exposure.

Biohacking Techniques

Often scores on the visual contract sensitivity (VCS) test decline for a few days after a particularly problematic mold exposure.

Detox also can drive down the VCS score.

Heart rate, heart rate variability or blood pressure often spike immediately upon exposure.

Other available health tracking measures include time spent in specific sleep stages (such as REM or deep sleep), motion, amount of perspiration, and skin temperature.

Inability to do math tends to be associated with mold toxin exposures (and particularly with exposures to the Mystery Toxin).

Trying to solve problems from a book of math puzzles or to count back from 100 in increments of 7 can provide indicators of the extent to which math ability is impaired.

The tendency of the skin to acquire dents as a result of hypoperfusion can be indicative of the presence of certain mold toxins (especially the Mystery Toxin).

Indentations from socks or other mildly constrictive clothing as a result of hypoperfusion may suggest that exposures have recently taken place.

The Living Clean in a Dirty World blog post "Using a Pulse Test to Detect Problematic Foods and Environments" may be helpful for those attempting to pursue avoidance with objective measurements.

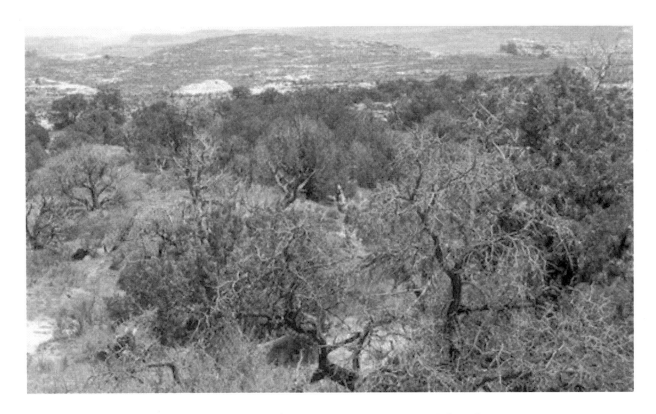

Colorado National Monument near Fruita, Colorado.

Chapter 34

The Power Curve

One of the peculiarities of dealing with mold toxins is that people tend to do better if they periodically can get clear of exposures.

Getting wholly clear of problematic toxins for discrete periods of time can be very helpful in terms of reducing their effects, even if exposures during the rest of the time are relatively high.

On the other hand, reducing the total amount of toxins to a level that is substantially lower - but still not low enough to really get clear – on a continual basis tends to be much less helpful.

In other words, managing the duration of the exposure to the toxins seems to be much more important than managing the total dose of the exposure.

Preemptively spending time in very clear areas with the goal of being able to tolerate more exposures during other times is referred to as "managing the power curve" or "balancing the books."

In many cases, people spend their time in clear areas doing recreational activities such as hiking or camping.

This can allow them to build up enough stamina to be able to better tolerate other necessary activities (such as working or taking care of family) in somewhat more problematic environments during the rest of the time.

Getting a Break

The observation that duration is especially important suggests that mold avoiders should focus energy on figuring out ways to get breaks from toxic exposures in places that are especially clear.

Spending even an hour getting really clear of inflammatory toxins in a very good environment can help the body to reset itself from ongoing toxic exposures, thus improving feelings of health regardless of whether toxic exposures the rest of the time remain unchanged.

Remaining in a good place for a more extended period of time can be even more helpful.

The Relative Shift

One of the most effective ways of moving permanently to a higher level on the power curve is to live a place with good air quality.

If the general air contains fewer problematic toxins, then this will remove a continual toxic exposure burden from the system.

As a result, getting clear will be easier.

Also as a result, tolerance of contaminated buildings or objects likely will be substantially higher.

This is what has been called the "relative shift": the exact same contaminated item may feel much less problematic in a good environment than it does in a bad environment.

The relative shift often manifests itself as the mold avoider being perplexed that a variety of objects all have "gone bad" for no apparent reason.

Often what has actually happened is that the air quality has gotten worse (for instance, due to an oncoming storm) and that the individual has become more affected by additional cross-contaminations as a result.

Sleep

Spending time in a particularly good environment while sleeping may be especially beneficial.

This appears to be at least in part because the body (especially the brain) tends to do much of its detoxification and repair work while sleeping.

Many mold avoiders have observed that their bodies detoxify much more readily when in a very good place than when in a less good place.

Sleeping in a very good place thus may allow the body to detoxify more efficiently.

Daytime Visits

In some cases, people have a hard time finding an ideal place in which to sleep on a regular basis.

For instance, the available options in a location where the individual needs to be may be less than pristine (and thus over tolerance) in terms of either the building or the outdoor air.

In that case, it can be helpful to find a nearby area that is particularly good and then to spend time there on a regular basis during the day.

For instance, many cities in the western US have wonderful wilderness areas only a short drive away.

Sometimes good spots can be present as little enclaves inside cities or suburban areas.

Often these are parks where few chemicals have been used; beaches; or spots at a higher elevation.

Any of these may have potential of feeling better than other locations even a few hundred yards away.

Once areas that are especially clear are identified, it may be helpful to spend as much time as possible there during the daytime hours.

Workplace Issues

For those mold avoiders who are able to work, finding a job in a building that is clear enough to feel really good may be a challenge.

Obviously, it would be best for mold avoiders not to work in a building that feels problematic for them at all.

Sometimes it is necessary for individuals to work in a somewhat problematic building in order to earn money or for other reasons, however.

If a building is substantially over tolerance, then it may not be realistic to think that measures such as breaking the response will be sufficient to compensate for wokplace exposures.

However, if a building is only somewhat over tolerance, making an effort to get really clear when not at work may be helpful in being able to tolerate the workplace better.

Activities could include leaving the building to go to a better place for an hour or more during the workday; sleeping in a particularly good environment; or spending weekends and holidays camping in really pristine places.

Filters and Masks

Individuals successful at improving their health through mold avoidance usually report that filtration devices and masks have played a limited role for them.

Although HEPA filters or other air filters may be capable of removing a high percentage of mold spores from the air, they are much less good at removing spore fragments and toxins.

Therefore, even if filters reduce the amount of toxicity in a building to some extent, they generally do not reduce it enough for those who have become hyperreactive to toxic mold to do well in those buildings.

Filters tend to be especially ineffective at addressing super toxin contaminations.

A common occurrence is for those periodically being exposed to Mystery Toxin to report initially that an air filter has been helpful, but then after a few days to find that the filtration unit itself has become the worst item in the house.

Typically when this occurs, just replacing the filter itself is not enough to solve the problem and the whole filtration machine will need to be discarded.

On the other hand, if the outside air is filled with a great deal of mildly toxic mold, filtration units may be of some help in reducing the amount to manageable levels.

For instance, the outdoor toxin (apparently Fusarium mold) associated with the usage of glyphosate has been reported to be filtered fairly effectively from the air with HEPA air filters.

While some successful mold avoiders do not use masks at all, others have reported that masks have been helpful in allowing them to spend relatively discrete amounts of time in buildings or other spaces that otherwise would have a negative effect on them.

Reports suggest that purchasing higher-quality masks and then changing the filters frequently may helpful.

As with home air filters, masks tend to work much better when regular mold toxins rather than super toxins are involved.

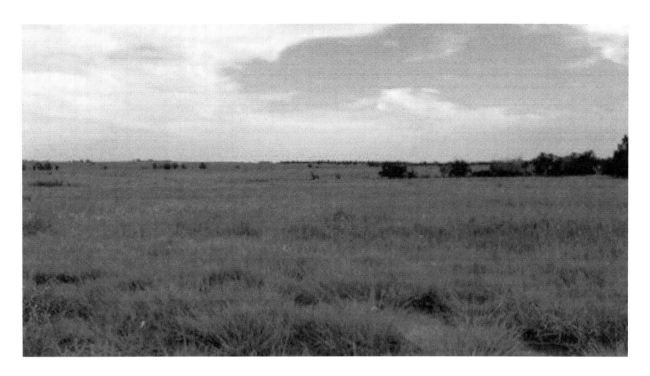

The Texas panhandle.

Chapter 35

Controlling Cross-Contamination

Learning to control cross-contamination is an extremely important part of successful practice of mold avoidance.

Toxic mold has the ability to cross-contaminate to a much larger extent than human-made chemicals do.

This means that items that have been exposed to moldy environments may become problematic enough to keep people who are hyperreactive to mold toxins totally sick.

In some cases those items may have the potential of cross-contaminating other items so that the latter are toxic enough to cause severe health symptoms in hyperreactive individuals.

Dust vs. Chemicals

Controlling cross-contamination becomes much easier when the actions of the spores and spore fragments are considered separately from the actions of the toxins.

Toxic mold spores are living things containing protein and also saturated with poison.

They are produced in a mold colony.

Dormant spores from the colony eventually are sent off into the air, where they float around for a while and then eventually settle on the floor or other flat surfaces.

In some cases, the spores remain whole, with the potential of forming a new colony if the right conditions are encountered.

In other cases, the spores disintegrate into spore fragments.

The toxic spores or toxic spore fragments mix with other dust in the environment.

When this toxin-laden dust comes into contact with an object, it has the tendency to stick to that object for a while.

Then later, the toxic dust particles may fall off that object and onto a different object.

As the toxic dust particles remain stuck to an object for an extended period of time, some of the toxin itself transfers to the object.

Tight vs. Loose Bonds

The bond between the dust particles and a particular object is quite loose.

Particles easily fall off some objects and then stick to other objects.

The bond between the toxin itself and the object is much stronger.

This results in some peculiarities in mold avoidance.

For instance, if an object has been exposed to an environment that contains a super toxin for an extended period of time, then generally that object will be extremely difficult or impossible to remediate.

The reason is because the super toxins themselves will transfer to the object, sticking very firmly to it.

On the other hand, if an object is exposed to an environment that contains a super toxin for a relatively short period of time, then generally that object will be much easier to remediate.

If the spores or spore fragments have been sticking to the object for only a short period of time, they generally will not have had much of a chance to transfer their toxin to the object.

If that is the case, then a quick rinse will be sufficient to remove the spores and spore fragments from the object and thus to resolve the problem.

The most problematic super toxins (Mystery Toxin and Hell Toxin) appear to have the ability to transfer to objects much more quickly than other mold toxins.

This is part of what makes them so problematic.

Still, insofar as there is going to be a chance of saving an object that is contaminated with those toxins, rinsing it quickly may have the best likelihood of success.

The Safe Space

At the core of dealing with cross-contamination is the establishment of a safe space.

The goal is to have a place to spend time (especially while sleeping) that is as free of problematic toxins as it can be.

For most people, the living space (whether it is a building, a vehicle or a tent) will be a designated safe space.

The sleeping area should be kept particularly clear.

Very likely when leaving the safe space to spend time in civilization, exposures to problematic toxins will occur.

For instance, buildings visited may have mold in them.

The outdoor air could have problematic toxins in it.

Cross-contaminations may be picked up by sitting on chairs.

Cross-contamination may affect the car, due to objects being transported in it.

Although spending time being exposed to problematic toxins may not be pleasant, health effects can be minimized by making sure that those toxins are not brought back to contaminate the safe space.

This is accomplished by rinsing everyone and everything that is suspected to be cross-contaminated before it enters the safe space, in order to remove the toxin-laden dust.

Once people and items are rinsed, they can enter the safe space with much less risk of cross-contaminating it.

Vehicles

Unless people are always driving around with a shower (such as in a truck camper), they invariably will find it necessary on some occasions to get into their vehicle after visiting problematic places without decontaminating.

In addition, vehicles may be exposed to toxins from the outside air or as a result of transporting contaminated possessions.

Since the inside of most vehicles is impossible to wash thoroughly, many people pursuing avoidance choose not to designate their vehicle as a safe space.

Rather, they do what they can to keep the vehicle from getting badly contaminated (including possibly covering the seats with towels that can be washed as needed) but nonetheless plan to decontaminate after each vehicle use before re-entering their safe space.

Types of Toxins

Certain toxins cross-contaminate much more than others.

Learning to immediately identify the toxins that are especially likely to cross-contaminate can be helpful in determining how much care needs to be taken to guard against them.

In general, while objects may become problematic as a result of being contaminated with regular mold toxin, only a very few super toxins seem to have the potential of transferring from object to object to enough of an extent to cause threats to the safe space.

Therefore, figuring out warning signals with regard to toxins that do and that do not cross-contaminate to a high extent can be helpful in reducing the amount of effort that control of cross-contamination requires.

Receiving Packages

Items received via delivery service may be at least as apt to cross-contaminate an environment as items obtained locally.

Therefore, treating all packages received with caution may be a good idea.

For instance, packages may be opened outside the living environment and their contents rinsed if necessary before integrating them into the living space.

Problem Items

Some items such as books cannot be rinsed and are often cross-contaminated.

Particular care should be taken with these objects to make sure that they are not contaminated with super toxins before integrating them into the safe space.

Electronics items can be particularly tricky because it sometimes is not evident that they are contaminated with particularly problematic toxins until they are turned on.

Certain laptop computers have been known to contaminate entire environments with Hell Toxin as soon as the fan goes on, for instance.

Thus, operating electronics items outdoors until it is ascertained that they are safe may be a good idea.

Groceries

Like any other item, groceries (including packaged goods as well as produce) have the potential of being cross-contaminated with especially problematic mold toxins.

A few very reactive individuals have noted having issues with certain grocery items.

So far, most mold avoiders have not found it necessary to rinse or carefully evaluate all grocery items before bringing them into the safe space of the home.

Those who are particularly reactive may consider carefully whether it would be prudent for them to do so, however.

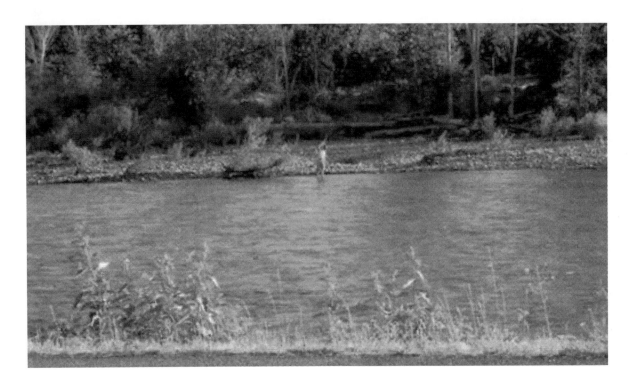

Fly fishing on the river in downtown Missoula, Montana.

Chapter 36

Decontamination

Subsequent to visiting problematic or suspect environments, it is important not to bring toxins encountered back into the designated safe space.

By decontaminating (showering and changing clothes) before re-entering the safe space, mold avoiders can substantially decrease the likelihood that problematic toxins will make their way into the safe space.

In addition, decontaminating quickly after a major hit can vastly reduce the negative effects of the exposure.

Mold avoiders also may find that they are sweating out problematic mold toxins through their skin and that they are bothered by these until they decontaminate.

Routine Decontamination

Many people choose to decontaminate routinely every time they return to their safe space after going out.

Typically, clothing is shed just inside the door.

If clothing is suspected as being contaminated with problem toxins, it can be immediately put into a bag for storage until it can be washed.

The bag will keep the items from shedding toxic dust into the safe space and contaminating it.

If the clothing is particularly contaminated, the bag may be placed outside the safe space until it can be dealt with.

Except for very bad contaminations in a small space (such as an RV), this may not be necessary for most people though.

The next step is to rinse or wash the body and hair thoroughly, so that any poisonous dust clinging to it is removed.

It usually is easiest to do this in a shower, but a sponge bath (with rinsing of hair) could suffice.

Use of chemicals or particularly harsh soaps have not been reported to be necessary for mold avoidance decontamination to be effective.

In fact, since some mold toxins (including Hell Toxin) have been reported to get worse when treated with chemicals, choosing the mildest soaps available may be a good idea.

Natural castile soap (such as Dr. Bronner's or Just So) can be a good choice.

Some mold avoiders state that soap containing charcoal, EDTA or other detoxifying agents has been helpful to them.

Although even just rinsing the hair may be effective at removing most cross-contaminations, some mold avoiders report certain shampoos to be especially effective.

Some mold avoiders also say that rinsing their sinuses can be helpful after exposures.

Mini Decontamination

Not infrequently, mold avoiders may inadvertently be hit by a bad environment that will have an immediate negative effect on them.

Especially when people are very reactive, the cross-contamination of hair and clothes from even a 30-second exposure to a bad building or encounter with a bad outdoor plume can make them increasingly sick until they decontaminate.

Ideally, a full shower would be immediately available for such incidents.

However, unless people are able to bring a shower with them everywhere that they go, there likely will be times when a shower is not immediately available.

In those instances, just rinsing the hair with water, wiping exposed skin (such as face and neck) with wet towels, and changing the shirt often can make an enormous difference.

Often this can be accomplished in the restroom of a fast food restaurant or other public establishment.

In warm weather outside of cities, just dumping a small bottle of water on the hair outdoors and changing the shirt in the car may be sufficient to stop the reaction.

Mini-decontaminations may be much easier with short hair than with long hair.

In some cases, individuals have reported that wearing a hat of some kind into suspect buildings and then removing the hat (and changing their shirt) afterwards is enough to stop a reaction without a need to rinse the hair.

Keeping the spare shirt or other clothing in a plastic bag will prevent it from getting inadvertently contaminated.

Generally, the mini-decontamination is followed by a full decontamination upon return home.

Hell Toxin

Reports suggest that Hell Toxin not only cross-contaminates more than other toxins, it also is less likely to fully wash off.

Epsom salt baths (or the use of Epsom salts as a body scrub) may be helpful in removing Hell Toxin from the body.

An exfoliator of some kind also may be helpful.

Chemicals of all sorts are reported to make Hell Toxin worse rather than remediating it.

A few reports suggest that vinegar can exacerbate the effects of the Hell Toxin as well.

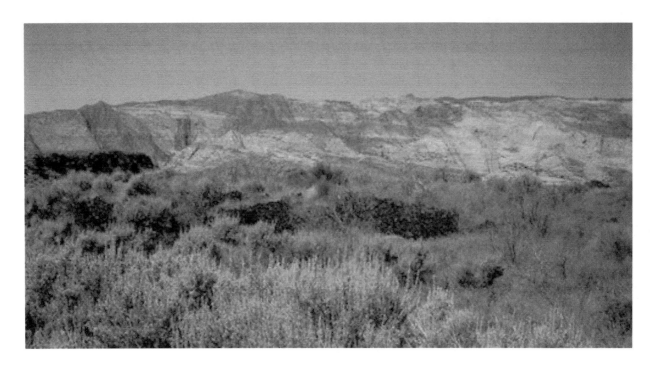

Snow Canyon State Park near St. George, Utah.

Chapter 37

Remediating Cross-Contaminations

Mold avoiders vary in terms of how much effort they put into remediating cross-contaminations.

Cross-contaminating toxic dust that contains spores and spore fragments is usually relatively easy to remove as long as an item can be washed with water (or at least wiped with a damp cloth).

The toxins that stick to objects are much more difficult to remove.

Remediating possessions that have long been in an environment problematic enough to make people feel very sick very often is an impossible task.

Many mold avoiders end up losing most or all of their previous possessions because remediating them is difficult or impossible.

People who are just starting avoidance also may make mistakes in terms of being exposed to toxins for longer than would be optimal.

After individuals get clear, they sometimes find that they begin detoxifying toxins that are difficult to remediate from clothing or bedding through their sweat.

Therefore, many mold avoiders become resigned to purchasing items - especially clothes - with the intention of using them only until they become too contaminated to be comfortable.

Other mold avoiders have put substantial amounts of time into trying a wide variety of alternatives to try to remediate their possessions.

Generally it has been found to be preferable to use agents that will gently remove the spores.

Killing the spores tends to prompt a toxic release that will make the item feel much worse and thus may be best avoided if possible.

If items can be rinsed with water, this is generally considered to be the best first step.

If problems then persist, other methods can be tried.

Following is a summary of a few options.

Altitude

The drop in barometric pressure from an increase in altitude generally causes a toxin release.

The cross-contaminated object will feel worse while at the higher altitude, but then often will feel better than it previously did when it is brought back down to the original altitude.

This remediation strategy can be especially helpful for RV's and cars that have been briefly hit by a plume of the Mystery Toxin.

The trip to altitude seems to loosen up the toxins, allowing them to be much more easily washed off surfaces.

Other kinds of objects may benefit from time spent at altitude as well.

Although larger changes in altitude may prompt the most dramatic results, even a relatively small change in altitude (such as a few hundred feet) may make a noticeable difference.

Altitude tends to be more effective than most other methods for remediating plastic or other porous items.

Sun

The UV light from the sun seems to have the ability to degrade mold toxins (including most super toxins) relatively well.

Bright sun (such as is present in the desert or at high altitude) tends to be more effective at this than less bright sun.

Artificial UV lights are reported to be much less effective than bright sun.

Remediation even from bright sunlight may take weeks or months for some toxins.

Badly contaminated items may take even more time.

Briefly contaminated items may benefit from being exposed to bright sunlight even for a few hours.

Plastic is reported to be more resistant to the effects of the sun than many other items.

Time

Cross-contaminations of even the worst toxins eventually fade away.

However, if items are badly cross-contaminated, it may be many years before they are usable again by those who are hyperreactive.

Objects are more likely to die down over time if they are wrapped loosely or left unwrapped rather than encased in plastic.

Storing objects in a hot, dry place may be optimally effective in getting them to die down faster.

Mold spores can sometimes remain intact and able to serve as the basis for new colonies for hundreds or even thousands of years.

If a mold was problematic enough to cause possessions to have to be stored for an extended period of time, then reintroducing its spores into a new environment is taking a risk that this same mold will establish itself again.

Washing items before putting them into storage (or before re-introducing remediated objects into the present environment) is thus advised.

Storing unwashed items in a damp environment may lead to additional mold growth, especially with some types of mold.

Heat

Mycotoxins are generally stable up to high temperatures, such as 500 degrees or more.

Some mold avoiders have reported success in remediating certain cross-contaminations with the use of a flamethrower blowtorch.

Obviously, this is a very dangerous method that can only be used safely on a very few cross-contaminated items such as those made of metal.

Metal pans (such as cast iron) may have the potential of being remediated by heating them to high temperatures on a stove.

This may cause a toxic release and thus preferably would be done outside, such as on a barbeque grill.

Probiotics

Probiotic bacteria are generally very good at neutralizing mycotoxins.

Homemade kefir seems especially effective, but effective microorganisms (EM-1) also may be helpful.

Reports suggest that insofar as an item still has spores on it, the bacteria will first kill the spores and make the item feel worse through the toxin release.

Eventually the microbes will degrade the toxin as well.

While it is impractical to soak most items in milk kefir, using it in RV holding tanks to control both mold growth and toxins has been reported as helpful.

Reports suggest that probiotics may be effective on Hell Toxin.

Ozone

Although ozone is inappropriate in itself to remediate buildings in which mold is growing, a number of mold avoiders have reported successfully using it to repair cross-contaminations of mold toxin.

Generally the amount of ozone needed in order to remediate cross-contaminations is a level that will harm electronics and certainly that is unsafe for humans to breathe.

The biggest success stories with ozone tend to come from isolating an object in a box or envelope and letting strong ozone run for an extended period of time (such overnight).

Occasionally individuals who are camping (especially in humid and non-pristine areas) report that small amounts of toxic mold may grow spontaneously on their tent, bedding or other items.

The periodic use of ozone may be especially appropriate for addressing this spontaneous mold growth.

As with probiotics, ozone will first cause the spores to release toxins (making things feel worse) prior to the toxin being degraded.

Longer periods of exposure thus may be more effective than shorter periods.

Degreasers

Vulpex is a commercial cleaner that is said by some mold avoiders to have the potential of removing most mold toxin contaminations.

Other caustic degreasers may be helpful for some contaminations as well.

Reports suggest that degreasers are not helpful for Hell Toxin contaminations.

Degreasers also have the potential of being offensive to those with chemical sensitivities and may be inappropriate to use on some types of items (including those made of cement, aluminum or certain other metals).

Vodka

Some mold avoiders report vodka (perhaps with grapefruit seed extract added) to be an effective general cleaner for cross-contaminations.

Essential Oils

Oils of various sorts (including the popular Thieves' Oil) may have the ability to degrade some mold toxins slightly.

Butter

Some mold avoiders report success at using butter (followed by washing with soap) to remove mold toxins from non-porous items.

Bleach

Soaking fabric items such as towels overnight in a strong bleach solution may be effective at resolving most contaminations.

Shorter exposures to milder bleach solutions tend to irritate the spores into releasing toxin and not resolve the problem.

Vinegar

Vinegar tends to irritate spores into releasing toxins without fixing the problem.

Vinegar has been reported to make Hell Toxin much worse.

Wash Water

Especially when Hell Toxin is involved, disposing of used wash water somewhere away from the living environment rather than pouring it on the ground may be a good idea.

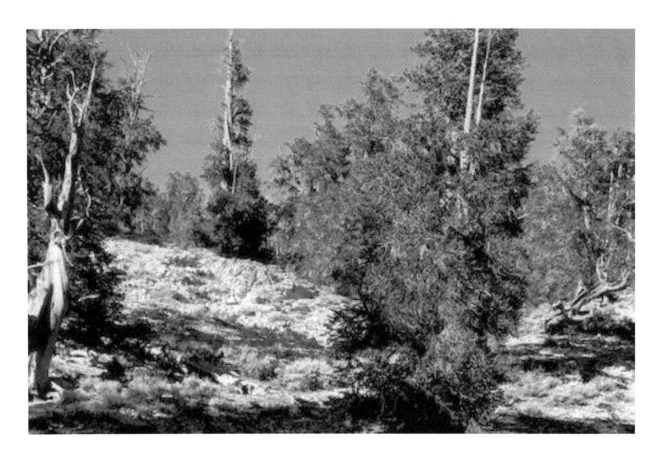

The Ancient Bristlecone Pine Forest near Bishop, California.

Chapter 38

Laundry

Laundry is a real challenge for mold avoiders.

The main problem is related to Hell Toxin, which has repeatedly been reported to "explode" in washing machines (and perhaps to grow in them).

Other toxins (including Mystery Toxin) can contaminate both washers and dryers as well.

In addition, automatic dryers take in large amounts of air from the immediate environment, with the clothing inside acting as a filter for the toxic mold or other contaminants present in the air.

Therefore, doing laundry in automatic machines is an activity that carries a substantial risk for mold avoiders.

Hand washing most is suggested.

Automatic Machines

A number of mold avoiders have reported permanently ruining their own washing machines as a result of washing items contaminated with small amounts of Hell Toxin.

These contaminated washing machines have subsequently permanently contaminated all other clothing that is washed in them.

In many cases, they have negatively affected the entire dwelling as well.

In almost all cases, no amount of effort has succeeded in remediating washing machines contaminated with Hell Toxin.

Therefore, if mold avoiders have an automatic machine that feels good to them, they may be best off using it only for items that they are sure have not been cross-contaminated with Hell Toxin.

For instance, providing that everyone in the household is decontaminating upon return to the house, items such as bedding, towels and nightclothes conceivably could be put through the washing machine.

Some mold avoiders soak items first and then see if they react to them.

If they do not react, they then put the items through their good machine to get them really clean.

Automatic dryers also have the potential of being cross-contaminated with particularly problematic toxins.

In some cases, dryers will die down from certain toxins (such as Mystery Toxin) after many months of constant use in a dry environment.

If the air has problem toxins in it, the automatic dryer will consolidate those toxins disproportionately on clothing or other items that are put through it.

If the washer becomes contaminated with Hell Toxin, the dryer very likely will become permanently contaminated as well.

Hand Washing

Doing laundry by hand takes some effort.

People who are still ill and who are doing laundry for a whole family may find this to be especially difficult.

However, the reports of mold avoiders who have had their lives turned upside down as a result of experiences with Hell Toxin suggest that it nonetheless may be worthwhile.

Many mold avoiders have reported that the Wonderwash is convenient and effective in getting clothing clean with minimal effort.

The Wonderwash has the advantage of agitating laundry with just a few turns of the handle, without the need for electricity.

It is especially appropriate for outdoor use, but also can be used inside.

A downside is that it takes up a fair amount of room in a car or RV.

A large sink, a bathtub, a bucket or a large plastic storage bin also may be appropriate for doing hand laundry.

For large items such as coats or sleeping bags, a plastic garbage can could be used.

For other methods of washing by hand, some people find a specialty plunger to be helpful for agitation.

If agitating or wringing without tools, plastic or rubber gloves could be considered.

One option to vastly speed up the drying of clothing, towels and sheets (and to allow those items to be dried hanging in an open closet) is a spin dryer.

However, for those camping, a spin dryer may not be appropriate since it requires electricity and also takes up a good bit of room in the car.

A clothes wringer is another possibility, though this will need to be mounted somewhere in order to be used.

A mop wringer attached to a bucket also may remove much of the water from clothing.

Other items to have on hand for laundry: clotheslines, bungee cords and clothespins.

Choosing clothing that dries quickly may make doing laundry by hand easier.

Laundry Detergent

Hell Toxin has been consistently reported as becoming more problematic when treated with any kind of modern chemical.

Vinegar also may exacerbate Hell Toxin.

As a preventative measure that may make it more likely that inadvertent Hell Toxin contaminations will be washed away without even being noticed, laundry detergent that is as natural as possible may be preferable.

For instance, one possibility could be a homemade laundry soap powder containing borax, washing soda and grated castile soap.

Dr. Bronner's liquid soap could be substituted for the grated soap.

Some people find oxy-type laundry products to be more tolerable in terms of chemical sensitivities than borax or washing soda.

Hydrogen peroxide may be effective for brightening whites without bleach.

Other natural laundry soaps not containing vinegar also might be appropriate.

Homemade kefir or effective microbes (EM-1) are an interesting idea for doing laundry since probiotics seem to be good at degrading mycotoxins.

It may be safer to rinse items to remove spores before treating with probiotics, however.

For stains, it may be safer to treat with an oxy-type product and then to wash the affected item separately than to use a stain-removing commercial detergent on everything.

Hell Toxin

Reports consistently suggest that Hell Toxin is difficult or impossible to remove from fabrics.

If a fabric item is causing substantial itching or burning, it may be best to just throw it away.

If an attempt is made at washing items contaminated with Hell Toxin, doing so one item at a time by hand is advised.

Water Contamination

Although the official government advice about cyanobacteria contaminations of water is that boiling does not help, a number of mold avoiders have stated that boiling tap water that they know to be contaminated with cyanobacteria toxin makes it feel better to them.

If tap water is suspected of being contaminated with cyanobacteria toxins, it might be worth boiling the water before using it for laundry.

Some mold avoiders boil large amounts of water on the stove on a regular basis, then store the boiled water for use in washing later on.

Another simple way to wash clothes in boiled water is to heat some water to boiling in a large pot, then turn off the heat and add a few garments when the temperature gets to the desired level.

Adding soap tends to complicate this method, but a bit of lemon could be used for disinfecting.

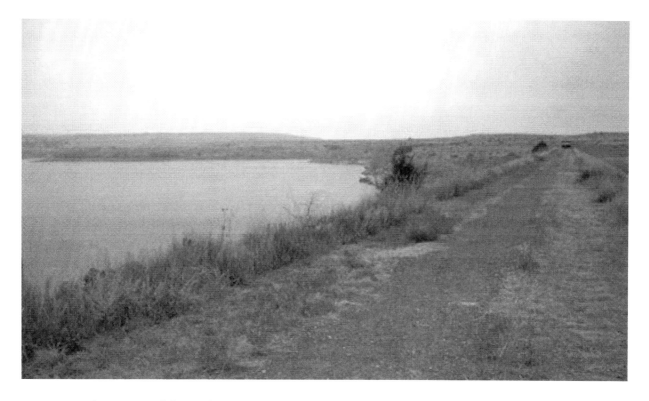

The Bosque del Apache National Wildlife Refuge near San Antonio, New Mexico.

Chapter 39

Outdoor Toxins

For the most part, even people who know that they are hyperreactive to mold toxins or other environmental agents tend to vastly underestimate the effect that outdoor toxins may be having on their well-being.

This is partly because unless they make a particular effort, many people (especially those who are ill) do not often visit a variety of locations.

Even when individuals travel to other places, they may attribute changes in how they feel to things such as being on vacation, travel stress, being in a different indoor environment, or post-exertional malaise.

Mold avoiders who have made a particular effort to test how they feel in different locations usually report that what has been called the "locations effect" has just as much of an impact on how they feel as indoor air quality does.

Therefore, especially for people who are very ill, considering the idea that outdoor toxins may be exerting an important influence may be worthwhile.

Following is a discussion of some outdoor airborne toxins that are fairly common and that seem to have a negative effect on many or all individuals who are hyperreactive to mold toxins.

More information can be found in the Paradigm Change blog post titled "Outdoor Toxins of Particular Importance to Mold Illness Patients."

Mystery Toxin

This particularly problematic toxin is discussed in Chapter 30.

Certain locations are affected particularly severely by this toxin.

In general, mold avoiders tend not to do well in those locations.

Toxin Associated with Agriculture

Certain agricultural areas are affected by an outdoor substance that has a particularly problematic effect on individuals who are hyperreactive to mold toxins.

Anecdotally, these areas tend to be places where the chemical herbicide glyphosate (Roundup) is used on crops.

Agricultural areas in the Midwest where corn or soybeans (both Roundup Ready crops) predominate can be especially affected, for instance.

Although some mold avoiders are reactive to agricultural chemicals as well as to biotoxins, this reactivity does not seem to be to the herbicide itself.

It may be that it is a reaction to the toxins made by Fusarium, a trichothecene-producing mold that has been shown in literature to grow to a particularly problematic extent in fields that have been treated with glyphosate.

Residential areas may be affected with a toxin that feels like this as well.

Locations that are affected by this toxin tend to feel better during winter months than summer ones.

Possibly this is because the cold and snow make the mold that is creating the toxin less present in the air.

This toxin seems to be similar in effects to the regular toxic mold (including regular Stachybotrys) present in many buildings.

Although this toxin cross-contaminates only mildly and can be washed out, living in an area where it grows can have a negative effect on those who are affected by it.

Air filters may be helpful in removing this toxin from the air.

Toxin Associated with Fire Retardants

This toxin can be difficult even for people who are successfully pursuing avoidance of mold in buildings to identify immediately.

Exposure tends to prompt only mild symptoms at first, such as the idea that the air does not feel clean or crisp.

Other initial exposure symptoms can be irritability or feelings of overwhelming sleepiness.

With continued exposures, those who are hyperreactive to toxic mold may be increasingly affected in negative ways.

This toxin tends to be much worse during the early evening hours than during the day.

Anecdotally, this substance seems to be especially present in areas that have previously been treated with fire retardants.

Reactions do not seem to be to the fire retardants themselves, but rather to some kind of microorganism growing in the wake of the fire retardant usage.

This toxin cross-contaminates relatively mildly and generally can be washed out, at least after relatively short exposures.

Air filters seem to be less effective with this kind of toxin than they are with the toxin associated with glyphosate.

Cyanobacteria Toxin

Airborne cyanotoxins such as BMAA are suspected as being a causal factor in amyotrophic lateral sclerosis (a fatal disease also known as ALS or Lou Gehrig's disease).

Individuals living in close proximity to lakes have been found to be especially likely to come down with ALS.

Anecdotally, many mold avoiders have reported finding outdoor cyanobacteria toxins to be problematic.

In some cases, these originate from a larger body of water like a lake or river.

Toxic cyanobacteria also can grow in a large enough quantity in ponds, creeks or ditches to be problematic to those hyperreactive to toxic molds.

Outdoor cyanotoxins in the outdoor air often manifest as a feeling of sleepiness or drunkenness.

Lack of coordination sometimes can result.

Feel-Good Locations

It is impossible to predict for sure whether a location will feel good in terms of outdoor toxins without visiting it.

In addition, locations can change in terms of how they feel over time.

However, here are some characteristics that tend to be associated with better locations for mold avoiders.

* **Pristine places.** Consistently, mold avoiders report that places that have been untouched by modern chemicals feel good to them.

* **Relatively undeveloped coastal areas.** Islands in the Caribbean or similar places often are reported as good locations even by those individuals with chronic multisystem disease who do nothing with regard to avoidance other than visit there on a vacation. Clean wind blowing off the ocean may be helpful, as may bright sunlight, negative ions and the presence of sand. Swimming also may be helpful in washing off cross-contamination brought from home.

* **High altitudes.** Problematic mold toxins tend to sink fairly readily toward the ground. This may account for why high altitudes tend to feel better than lower ones (provided

that large amounts of problem toxins are not emanating from those high-altitude places). Even a small altitude change, such as a few hundred feet, can make an enormous difference in some locations.

* **Remote desert environments.** Although some desert cities can be just as problematic as cities in other locations, more remote desert areas often feel good to those pursuing mold avoidance.

* **Green areas.** Provided that an area hasn't been treated with chemicals, the presence of plants can make a location feel better. Even a small green space, such as a city park, often can feel better than the area surrounding it.

* **Sunlight.** UV rays tend to neutralize mold toxins. This may explain why all things being equal, sunnier places tend to feel better than less sunny ones.

* **Sand.** Desert areas with a great deal of sand have been reported as feeling especially good to some mold avoiders.

Following are some factors that mold avoiders report tend to be associated with problem locations.

* **Cities.** It is a rare metropolitan area that feels really good to those pursuing mold avoidance. An exception may be when frequent fast winds blow local toxicity away.

* **Highly populated areas.** Even outside of cities, regions that are more highly populated can be problematic for mold avoiders. In the US, locations west of the Mississippi River are on average much clearer than ones in the more populated half of the country east of it.

* **Chemicals.** The environmental presence of virtually any kind of manmade chemical may create the conditions for mold avoiders to feel worse in a particular location, even if individuals are not hyperreactive to the chemicals themselves. Particularly problematic chemicals may include industrial solvent spills, fire retardants, and agricultural chemicals such as glyphosate.

* **Poor air circulation.** If a problematic area is located in a place where high mountains on one or more sides prevent good air flow, toxins may be more likely to remain stuck in that area rather than blowing away. Cities located in a basin (with mountains on all sides) may be particularly affected.

* **Humid areas.** Humidity does not seem to be a big problem for most mold avoiders in itself, provided that the area is pristine. High humidity does tend to compound the problems in polluted areas, however. (Individuals who have become reactive to all

molds rather than only to toxic molds may have difficulties in even pristine humid areas.)

Avoiding Outdoor Toxins

As is the case with indoor toxins, successful avoidance of outdoor toxins largely depends on the ability to identify the toxins upon immediate exposure to them.

Even for experienced mold avoiders, some of these toxins are not immediately noticeable in the outdoor air.

In addition, outdoor air in a particular location very often will be fine much of the time and then become problematic only periodically.

Often people focus on a variety of other exposure possibilities such as cross-contamination before considering that outdoor exposures could be the problem.

Avoiding outdoor toxins effectively involves taking into consideration the idea that locations may vary substantially over time, as a result of time of day or weather factors.

If the Mystery Toxin is suspected, then purchasing a barometric pressure monitor may be helpful when considering whether symptoms might be related to atmospheric shifts in problematic places.

Noting that symptoms tend to emerge at night is suggestive of the toxin associated with fire retardants.

Matching wind direction and speed with symptoms can provide information about the source points of the exposure.

Keeping track of these factors can make it easier to predict whether and when a particular area is likely to feel problematic in the future.

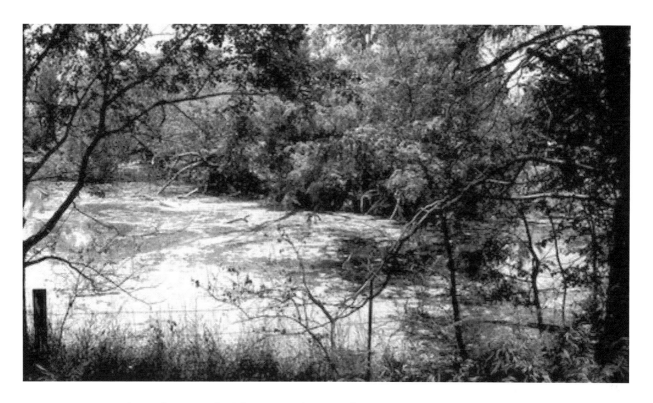

A creek covered with non-toxic cyanobacteria in La Crosse, Kansas.

Chapter 40

Water Contamination

Some cyanobacteria and other aquatic microorganisms have the ability to make toxins that are problematic for those individuals who are hyperreactive to toxic mold.

As described in Chapter 39, these toxins can be a problem in terms of inhalation of the air in certain places.

In locations where tap water is obtained from bodies of water contaminated by these microorganisms, the toxins also can be present in the tap water supply.

Some mold avoiders state that these toxins are not only a problem with regard to drinking the contaminated water, but also with regard to using it for washing.

Problematic Locations

A first step in considering whether the tap water might be an issue in a particular location is to look into the source of the water supply.

This information is generally available on the website of the local water department.

If water is obtained from underground sources and stored in tanks, it is much less likely to be contaminated with cyanobacteria toxin than if it is obtained from rivers or lakes.

Not all water that is obtained from or stored in rivers or lakes is contaminated with these kinds of toxins, however.

Some of these bodies of water are free of cyanobacteria in general or host only the non-toxic kind.

In addition, if water is obtained from a deeper part of a lake, cyanobacteria toxins may be less of an issue than if the water is obtained from an area of the lake closer to the surface or from a river.

In most locations, the extent to which cyanobacteria toxins are a problem in tap water varies over the course of the year.

Summer months often are particularly problematic.

Although online materials from water departments very often mention the extent to which the tap water supply contains cyanobacteria, information on whether the cyanobacteria involved are toxin producers generally is not provided.

Although specialized filtration technology is available to remove cyanobacteria toxins from water, the vast majority of water departments have not purchased it.

Effects on Mold Reactors

Contamination of drinking water supplies with aquatic biotoxins may have anything from a mild effect to a severe effect on people whoa are hyperreactive to mold toxins.

The strength of the effect may vary based on the amount of toxin present, the exact type of toxin present, and the degree of hyperreactivity.

Occasionally, toxins present in the tap water may be problematic enough to qualify as super toxins.

In cases when stronger toxins or a greater quantity of toxins are present in tap water, the effects may be obvious.

In other cases, exposures to the milder cyanotoxins may push mold avoiders further down the power curve, making them more reactive to other exposures.

Washing with Contaminated Water

Water that is contaminated with cyanotoxins can be problematic regardless of whether it is ingested or used for washing.

Using contaminated water for showering or washing clothing may leave a residue that has the potential of being just as problematic to mold avoiders as drinking the water.

Even using the water for washing dishes or flushing toilets may have the potential of having a negative effect on some particularly reactive mold avoiders.

Cyanotoxins are reported to have similar effects regardless of whether the exposure is through tap water or directly from lakes, ponds or streams.

Typical symptoms are inflammation, interference with cognitive function, drunken feelings and declines in coordination.

Addressing Water Problems

One strategy with regard to this problem is to live in a location where the tap water is obtained from underground sources that do not have problematic toxins.

That may not always be possible, however.

Putting pressure on the local water department to purchase filtration that is effective on these toxins conceivably could solve the problem as well.

Especially subsequent to tap water contamination with cyanobacteria in some locations (such as Toledo, Ohio) receiving major media publicity, water departments may be more receptive to the idea of investing in this technology than they used to be.

Insofar as one must live in a place with constantly or periodically contaminated tap water, here are a few measures that might effectively address the problem.

The drinking water issue may be relatively easily solved through the use of bottled spring water.

Of course, this is expensive and less preferable for environmental reasons.

Most home filtration systems do not remove cyanotoxins from the water.

Reverse osmosis (RO) possibly may remove these toxins from the water, but RO systems are expensive and cumbersome for treating all tap water used.

A few mold avoiders have reported that boiling water prior to using it seems to resolve the contamination problem for them.

Boiling water contaminated with cyanotoxins releases those toxins into the air, meaning that good ventilation needs to be present in order to use this strategy.

While boiling enough water for routine showering, clothes washing or other purposes takes a considerable amount of work, some mold avoiders have found it to be helpful enough to be worth doing.

Other mold avoiders have reported purchasing distilled water from grocery stores or other commercial vendors and using it for laundry or washing.

Another alternative that some individuals have reported to be effective in reducing their exposure enough to make a difference is showering in regular tap water, then rinsing hair and face with bottled or boiled water.

Part 5

HEALING

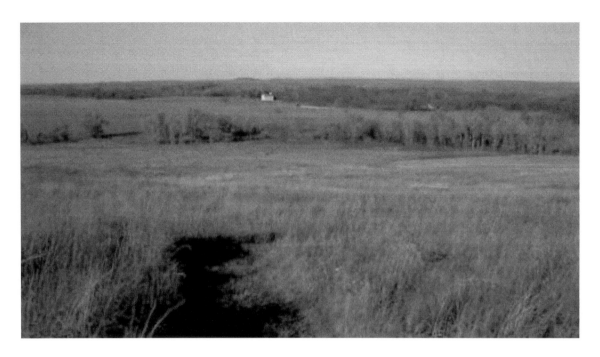

Tallgrass Prairie National Preserve in eastern Kansas.

Chapter 41

Compensating for Exposures

One of the first things that many people do after realizing the extent of their hyperreactivity is to consider ways to try to reduce the effects that exposures have on them.

Over the long run, it may be that detoxifying and repairing the system is the most effective way to reduce the extent to which toxic exposures are problematic.

Unfortunately, this can take years to accomplish with available tools.

In the meantime, even a small amount of reduction in the hyperreactivity component of the illness can make a big difference in quality of life.

Following is a discussion of some interventions that mold avoiders have reported to be helpful with regard to reducing their reactivity in the shorter term.

Note that while some of these treatments can be helpful for individuals who are less severely ill and getting significant exposures to problematic environments, it is not suggested that those individuals use them as a way to avoid having to reduce their exposures.

Insofar as susceptible people continue to be exposed to high levels of problematic toxins, their reactivity should be expected to continue to increase over time until these kinds of stopgap fixes cease working.

For people who are starting to show signs of illness, checking carefully for environmental exposures is important in order to avoid acquiring a more serious version of the illness.

Once this is done, interventions such as the following ones can be pursued.

Breaking the Response

As described in Chapter 34, spending part of the time in a pristine environment can help the body to tolerate somewhat more toxic exposures the rest of the time.

Maintaining a pristine safe space in a place with good outdoor air (or regularly spending time in a very good place during the daytime hours) can make a big difference in terms of being able to tolerate exposures during the rest of the time.

The "Epo Effect"

Some people have reported that exercising at an altitude at least a bit higher than their accustomed location can have a remarkably immediate effect in terms of helping them to get clear of inflammatory effects of toxins.

This is hypothesized to be related to the effects of erythropoietin ("epo"), a hormone that controls red blood cell production.

In order for this to work, the environment where the exercise is done needs to be clear of problematic toxins.

In addition, for those with exercise intolerance, the exercise needs to be kept at a pace that does not prompt a high heart rate to occur.

The positive effects (including decreases in reactivity) often are said to last a day or two after the exercise.

While it may be that exercising at a comparatively high altitude can be especially helpful, some people have stated that exercising at a moderate pace at any altitude can give them a boost as well.

Cold

Exposing agricultural animals to relatively low environmental temperatures has been shown in the literature to reduce the damage caused by mycotoxins.

A few mold avoiders have reported that ice baths, cold showers or cool living environments have the ability to decrease their reactivity and improve their feelings of health.

Even brief exposure to cold (such as may be obtained by alternating hot and cold water in the shower) possibly may be beneficial for this purpose.

Coffee Enemas

Coffee enemas appear to work primarily by removing toxins from the liver and gall bladder.

Many mold avoiders report them to be helpful in recovering more quickly from mold hits.

Diet

A clean diet that is low in mycotoxins as well as in chemicals may have the potential of reducing toxic stress on the system and thus allowing reactivity to environmental toxins to be a little less.

Paleo diets (especially the one advocated by Dave Asprey of the Bulletproof Executive) tend to be low in mycotoxins.

A diet heavy in raw foods may be helpful in reducing oxidative stress and thus possibly in decreasing reactivity.

Those who are reactive to gluten may find that eliminating it from their diets allows them to tolerate a little more environmental toxic exposure.

Experimenting with testing for other food reactivities and eliminating those that cause problems may be helpful as well.

Increasing Blood Volume

This is routinely suggested by ME/CFS doctors a way to combat the orthostatic intolerance (OI) suffered by many individuals with chronic multisystem illness.

It usually involves adding extra electrolytes (such as salt and potassium) to the diet and then drinking enough water to keep well-hydrated.

Certain medications such as Florinef may be helpful for this as well.

Because OI is often triggered by mold exposures and causes a variety of different negative effects, increasing blood volume may be helpful for people to remain somewhat more functional even when being exposed.

It does not serve as protection against other damage (such as harm to the brain or intestines) resulting from toxic exposures, however.

Vitamin C

One of the main ways that Stachybotrys causes systematic damage is via oxidative stress.

Other biotoxins deliver oxidative stress as well.

If people with chronic illness are living in a home with large amounts of problematic mycotoxins, it will be hard to correct for it with any sort of treatment.

In a better environment, treatments that counter the effects of oxidative stress generated by smaller amounts of mycotoxins possibly may be helpful.

One of the most successful of these seems to be Vitamin C.

Vitamin C IV's seem to be especially effective, though it usually is considered a good idea to start at a low dosage and then consider raising the amount slowly.

Any Vitamin C that the body does not immediately use changes into hydrogen peroxide.

While this can be effective at killing pathogens, if pursued too aggressively it has the potential of causing a Herxheimer reaction.

Oxidative stress from hydrogen peroxide also has been shown to act synergistically with Stachybotrys toxin to create much more damage to human cells.

Many mold avoiders state that other forms of Vitamin C also may be helpful for countering oxidative stress from exposures.

The chewable, buffered and lyposomic forms have received particularly good reports.

Rectal delivery may be more effective than oral.

Curcumin

This is another natural anti-inflammatory supplement that has been reported by some mold avoiders as being helpful at reducing the effects of mold exposures.

Curcumin is the same thing as turmeric, which may be used in cooking.

Probiotics

Stachybotrys toxins are much more damaging when combined with LPS, a substance manufactured by certain pathogenic gut bacteria and certain environmental bacteria.

Therefore, working to decrease dysbiosis in the gut may be helpful in lowering reactivity.

One way to accomplish this is to focus on trying to increase the amount of good bacteria in the gut, since this tends to be inadequate in chronic multisystem disease.

Freshly made probiotic foods (such as kefir, yogurt or sauerkraut) have been reported to be much better at replenishing good bacteria in the gut than probiotic capsules.

Probiotic foods have the potential of creating a die-off and may be best started slowly.

Individuals sensitive to histamine sometimes report negative effects from certain probiotic foods, and so this suggestion may not be appropriate for everyone.

VIP

Vasoactive intestinal peptide (VIP) is a regulatory neuropeptide produced naturally in the human body.

Mold illness patients tend to produce less of this substance (as well as less of another regulatory neuropeptide called MSH) than healthy people do.

Supplementation of VIP is available by prescription and is reported in the literature to have a number of positive effects on mold illness patients.

A few mold avoiders have reported that VIP has been somewhat helpful in decreasing their reactivity and in helping them to feel better.

Glutathione

Some mold avoiders state that supplemental glutathione can help to compensate for a toxic mold hit.

Nebulized glutathione is often used for this purpose, but other forms of glutathione may be helpful as well.

Low-Dose Naltrexone

This is an opioid receptor antagonist that serves as an immunomodulator.

A few mold avoiders have suggested that it has helped them to feel better in general and reduced their reactivity a bit.

Cannabis

Some mold avoiders report finding marijuana to be effective in increasing their resilience to mold hits.

Since marijuana growing operations have been reported to be contaminated with large amounts of mold (including toxic mold), quality issues should be considered.

Cannabis should not be used simultaneously with low-dose naltrexone.

Antivirals

Several people have reported that the use of antiviral medications targeted at herpes family viruses has been successful at lowering their reactivity a bit.

These medications may be easier to use with less die-off in a really good environment.

Antibiotics

A number of mold avoiders have stated that taking doxycycline or similar antibiotics has helped to lower their reactivity to a noticeable extent.

Again, there may be less of a die-off and more effectiveness of the medications in a really good environment than a less good one.

Beta Blockers

Some individuals have found beta blockers to be helpful with regard to the orthostatic intolerance associated in particular with exposures to the Mystery Toxin.

Beta blockers have not been reported to help with the many other types of symptoms associated with exposures to this toxin, however.

Insofar as individuals remain clear of the Mystery Toxin, the usefulness of beta blockers has the potential of dissipating relatively quickly.

Thus, the continued need for beta blockers may be a clue that exposures to this problematic toxin are still being experienced.

Ampligen

Ampligen is an intravenously administered immunomodulator that binds to the TLR-3 receptors.

It may have the ability to provide some protection against trichothecene mold toxins, which have been found to affect TLR-3 in a negative way.

A subset of very ill ME/CFS patients have been reported to benefit from this drug.

Reports about Ampligen suggest that it might be helpful with regard to lowering the reactivity of mold avoiders enough for them to be able to lead a more normal life.

This could be especially useful during the early stages of avoidance, when a desirable goal may be to get clear enough to detoxify substantially (thus hopefully lowering reactivity into the future).

Unfortunately, Ampligen is an experimental drug available only through a few doctors - almost all of them located in locations that are quite problematic.

The out-of-pocket cost (up to $50,000 a year) is an additional barrier.

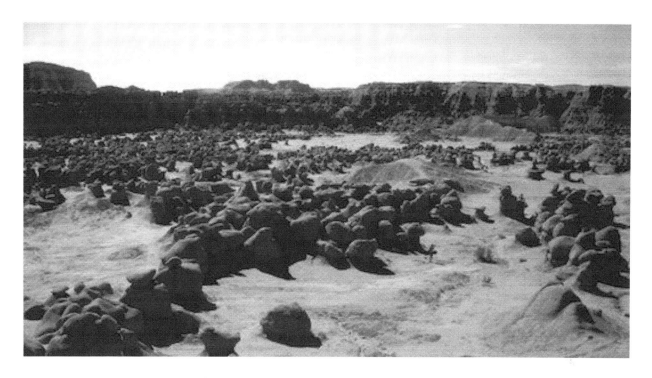

Goblin Valley State Park in northeastern Utah.

Chapter 42

Detoxification

A high percentage of those mold avoiders who have managed to lower their reactivity and reclaim a more normal life give much of the credit to detoxification.

Successful detoxification can require a substantial amount of work and a considerable amount of thought, however.

Getting Clear

Detoxification generally occurs much more readily and with much less pain and suffering when the body is really clear of environmental exposures.

Even if it is not possible to live permanently in an extremely good place, spending an extended period of time in one for detox purposes may be worth considering.

Types of Toxicity

People who are reactive to mold very often have large amounts of stored heavy metals and chemicals as well as mold toxins in their systems.

Removal of any of these substances seems to have the potential of generating improved health and decreased mold reactivity.

Detoxification Channels

Individuals with mold illness often suffer from impairments of a variety of different detoxification channels.

In order for successful detoxification to occur, all of these impairments need to be addressed.

Astounding Amounts

Anecdotally, virtually all of those mold avoiders who have managed to lower their reactivity enough to move toward living a normal life state that they were astounded by how toxic their systems were once they managed to create the conditions by which toxins could be removed effectively.

Mold avoiders who have not experienced this phenomenon and who are having a hard time lowering their reactivity may want to consider whether they may be able to address detoxification blockages that are preventing them from clearing toxins successfully.

Stone-Age Tools

Tools currently available for detoxification are almost all extremely primitive.

Despite the increasing evidence that toxicity is largely responsible for a wide variety of modern diseases, modern medicine remains focused much more on killing pathogens, tweaking systems and surgery.

Perhaps at some point in the future, researchers' attention will turn more toward the idea that better detoxification tools might be helpful to people whose chronic health conditions are not being effectively treated in other ways.

Emotional Aspects

Many patients have reported that detoxification can prompt strong emotional reactions.

This may be because these neurotoxins have the ability of blocking normal emotional experiences from being fully processed.

A few mold avoiders have reported that actively processing emotions (such as through psychotherapy) can be helpful in promoting detoxification.

Much more often, mold avoiders report that promoting detox through physical approaches prompts emotional release that can be painful in the short-term but that eventually leads to a happier and healthier emotional state.

Taking Breaks

Especially when pursued aggressively, detoxification tends to be very hard on the body.

Periodically taking breaks to allow the system to recover may be important.

Supporting the system with a particularly good diet tends to be reported as much more helpful by people who are pursuing mold avoidance and actively detoxifying their systems than it is by those individuals with chronic multisystem disease who are not avoiding mold.

Although nutritional supplements occasionally are reported as being somewhat helpful, acquiring nutrients through food (especially large amounts of organic produce and high-quality fats) usually is reported as much more effective.

Comprehensive Approaches

* **Mold and Environmental Illness Practitioners.** Medical or naturopathic doctors often use a wide variety of approaches to detoxification in their practices. These may include avoidance, nutritional supplements, saunas, chelation, hormonal regulation, binders, dietary counseling, energy work, and body work.

* **Gerson Therapy.** Gerson (a controversial cancer treatment) has been reported by a number of chronic multisystem illness patients as having been intensely detoxifying and generating major improvements in their conditions. This is a labor-intensive diet program involving large amounts of fresh juice, cooked and raw vegetables, coffee enemas, castor oil (taken by mouth and in enemas), and a few supplements.

* **Methylation-Oriented Approaches.** A number of individuals with myalgic encephalomyelitis have reported experiencing intensely detoxifying experiences and long-term health gains after consulting individually with Amy Yasko, a biochemist and N.D. who specializes in methylation issues in autism. More simplified approaches (such as those proposed by Martin Pall or the late Rich van Konynenburg) also have reported as being helpful, though possibly more so for chemical sensitivities than mold hyperreactivity.

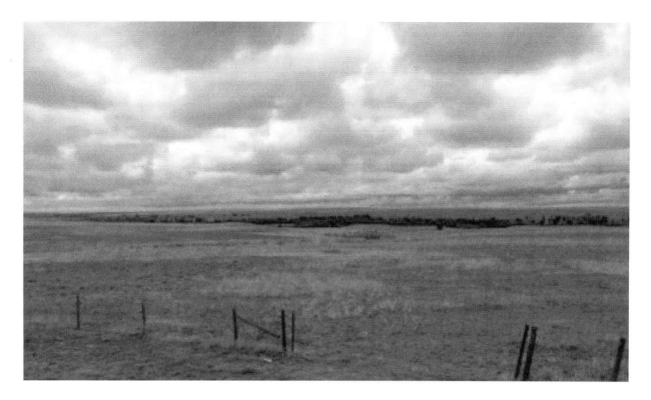

Comanche National Grasslands in southeast Colorado.

Chapter 43

Detoxification: Cells

One problematic issue for people who are trying to recover from chronic multisystem disease is that the toxins may become stuck in the cells.

People who have this issue often will not feel like their bodies are especially toxic, because the toxins will mostly be sequestered away.

Those sequestered toxins may be less overtly damaging than toxins that are loose in the system, but they nonetheless appear to be a major contributor to chronic health symptoms and hyperreactivity.

The experiences of many mold avoiders suggest that detoxification from the cells is much less likely to take place when people are in an environment that is over tolerance for them.

The working theory is that the system is trying to protect itself by releasing the toxins only in places where the current exposures are relatively low.

Even in a very good environment, the release of toxins from the cells may be suboptimal for some people.

Cellular Detox

Following are some approaches that have been reported as helpful in increasing detoxification at the cellular level.

* **Getting clear.** Even people who already are pursuing avoidance fairly successfully often are surprised to find that spending an extended period of time in a really pristine place can speed up detoxification from the cells substantially.

* **Supplements.** Certain nutritional supplements (including those related to methylation or treatment of pyroluria) may be useful in promoting detoxification at the cellular level. Some of these may include methyl folate (an activated form of folic acid), P-5-P (an activated form of B6), hydroxycobalmin or methylcobalmin (forms of B12), niacin, other B vitamins, zinc, selenium, iodine and lithium.

* **Phosphatidyl choline.** Some researchers suggest that problems with cell membranes can impede detoxification and that phosphatidyl choline (in oral or IV form) can help to address these.

* **Healthy fats.** High amounts of dietary fats such as coconut oil, butter (containing butyrate), fish oil and flax oil have been cited as helpful in allowing toxins to be purged at the cellular level.

* **Produce.** A diet with large amounts of fruits and vegetables (possibly including fresh juices or green smoothies) also can be helpful in promoting detoxification from the cells by providing the body with the nutrition that it needs in usable forms.

* **Infrared sauna.** Infrared light penetrates deep into the tissues and (provided that individuals are relatively clear) may have a loosening effect on toxins stored in the cells.

* **Electrolytes.** The Gerson Therapy (a controversial treatment for cancer that has been reported to be effective by a few ME patients) has as one of its tenets the idea that a diet that is very high in potassium and very low in sodium may be successful in forcing toxins to be released from the cells.

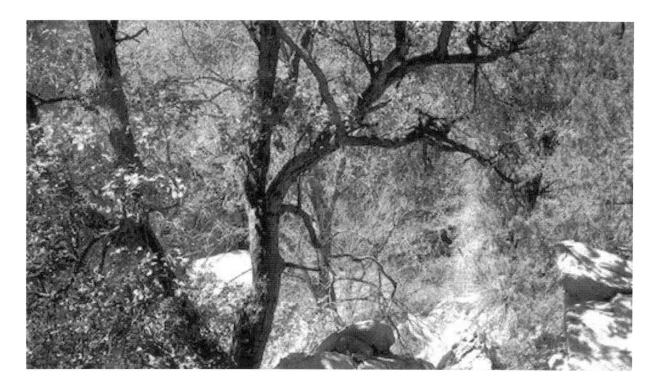

The Gila Wilderness in northwestern New Mexico.

Chapter 44

Detoxification: Drainage

Once toxins are released from the cells, they make their way to the detoxification organs through the lymphatic system.

In many patients with chronic multisystem disease, the flow of toxic material to and through the lymphatic system may be impeded.

This appears to be at least partially the result of the fascia (which is supposed to be soft and flexible) becoming tight and gummy.

Adhesions of the fascia can push down on tissues and lymph vessels, impeding flow of toxins from the system.

Fibromyalgia-type pain and brain inflammation can result.

Although this blockage of flow can occur throughout the body, it may be especially problematic when occurring at the base of the skull since this can impede the removal of toxins from the brain.

In addition, if the lymph is laden with toxins, it may become thicker and thus have more difficulty moving through the lymph vessels.

Unfortunately, getting to a pristine location has not necessarily been reported to fix drainage problems.

In fact, a number of patients have reported drainage to be more of an obvious problem in a good environment, presumably because the toxins that are being released from the cells are getting backed up in the system.

Promoting Drainage

Following are some interventions that have been reported by mold avoiders to be helpful in promoting drainage.

* **Neural therapy.** Small amounts of procaine are inserted with a fine needle into painful areas where adhesions are believed to be present. This requires finding a practitioner trained in the technique.

* **Bodywork.** This could include such things as massage, chiropractor treatments, cranial sacral or acupuncture.

* **Exercise.** Yoga, tai chi or similar exercises can be especially effective at addressing fascia issues and promoting drainage. Walking, swimming or other mild exercise may be helpful as well.

* **Heat.** Especially when combined with exercise or bodywork, heat may be helpful in improving fascia issues and lymphatic drainage.

* **Probiotics.** The use of fermented foods (such as homemade kefir, yogurt or sauerkraut) has been reported to have a positive effect on the fascia and thus on lymphatic drainage. A few reports suggest that certain packaged probiotics (such as Three Lac) also may be effective for some people.

* **Dietary changes.** Diets designed to correct dysbiosis in the gut - such as Paleo diets designed for autoimmune patients - may be helpful in addressing drainage issues.

* **Homeopathic remedies.** A number of homeopathic remedies state that they promote drainage. Natrum Sulphuricum is a remedy classically associated with damp buildings that has been reported by at least one mold avoider as being helpful for facilitating drainage from the brain.

* **Lymph cleansing herbs.** Certain herbs such as burdock appear to have the ability to thin the lymph, thus allowing it to move more easily through the lymph vessels.

* **Enzymes.** These could include enzymes from raw produce (such as juice) or from supplements (such as Wobenzym, lumbrokinase, nattokinase or serrapeptase).

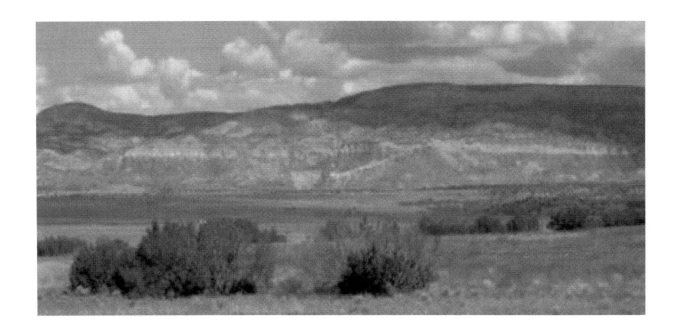

Abiqui, New Mexico.

Chapter 45

Detoxification: Liver, Gall Bladder & Kidneys

Prior to pursuing mold avoidance, the liver and kidneys often do not seem to be a particular problem in most patients with chronic multisystem disease.

This may be because the diastolic dysfunction in the disease (caused by a lack of energy in the heart) impedes the flow of toxins into the liver.

Once individuals become freer from toxic mold exposures, there tends to be less need for the body to reduce oxidative stress (known to exacerbate the damage done by certain mold toxins) by downregulating energy production in the heart and in the rest of the system.

Toxins thus may be more likely to flow into the liver from the system, as a result of the diastolic dysfunction being improved.

In addition, in a clearer environment, more toxins may be released from the cells and eventually make their way to the liver.

Therefore, stress on the liver may be more likely to occur when pursuing avoidance than it was while living in a problematic environment.

The gall bladder tends to be an especially problematic organ for many individuals who are being affected by toxic mold or are pursuing mold avoidance.

Often it fills up with black sludge and is removed by surgeons (who invariably express in amazement that they "never saw anything like this before").

Insofar as detox is going well, both the liver and the gall bladder will be under significant stress.

Kidneys may be under stress as well.

Supporting Detox Organs

Considering proactive interventions to keep detoxification organs functioning as optimally as possible may be worthwhile.

* **VIP.** Insofar as diastolic dysfunction (manifested by continued experience of orthostatic intolerance) has not yet been corrected, vasoactive intestinal peptide (VIP) may be helpful in improving the flow of toxins through the liver.

* **Coffee enemas.** These appear to be useful in purging toxins from the liver and gall bladder. Many mold avoiders report benefiting from coffee enemas, with some utilizing multiple coffee enemas per day at some points in their detoxification efforts.

* **Foods.** Foods that are reported to support the liver include bitter greens (such as dandelion), beets, artichokes and garlic. Foods that are said to be good for the kidneys include cruciferous vegetables, radishes, asparagus, garlic, onions, red bell peppers and berries of all types (especially cranberries).

* **Herbs.** A variety of herbs may be helpful for supporting the liver. These include bupleurum, dandelion root, silymarin, yellow dock and peppermint. Uva ursi, nettle, parsley and horsetail are amongst those herbs said to be helpful for the kidneys.

* **Acupuncture.** Traditional Chinese Medicine is reputed to be especially effective at supporting the liver. It may be helpful for kidneys as well.

* **Gall bladder cleanse.** Although the efficacy of gall bladder or liver cleanses is disputed, a number of mold avoiders report having benefited from doing them. These cleanses usually consist of drinking a good bit of apple juice over the course of a day, then following it with a combination of citrus juice and olive oil. Epsom salts or other laxatives are optional.

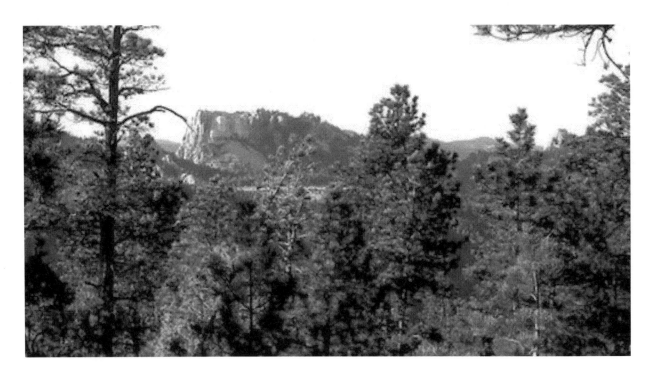

Mt. Rushmore in southwestern South Dakota.

Chapter 46

Detoxification: Intestinal Tract

The intestinal tract (especially the small intestine) is one of the systems of the body known to be most negatively affected by exposures to trichothecenes.

Insofar as these toxins pass through the digestive tract on the way out of the body, the small intestine may be damaged by them.

Especially for people with genetic susceptibilities, some toxins may have the tendency to be reabsorbed back into the system rather than passing through the intestinal tract and out of the body.

Individuals with chronic multisystem disease generally have dysbiosis in their intestinal tract.

This may include insufficient numbers of good bacteria and substantial amounts of undesirable pathogens of all sort.

Tapeworms and other worms that live in the small intestine have the ability to sequester heavy metals.

These intestinal parasites may compromise health when alive, but killing them has the potential of causing severe systemic damage due to the release of those dangerous metals.

Biofilms often contain heavy metals and provide protection to a wide variety of pathogens that may live in the digestive tract.

Intestinal permeability ("leaky gut") may be a direct effect of trichothecenes passing through.

Insofar as mold toxins must pass through the gut on their way out of the system, helping them to move through quickly may be worth some consideration.

Abdominal adhesions appear to be related to fibromyalgia.

Adhesions occur when the internal organs (especially the small intestines or the uterus) become dysfunctional due to the fascia becoming sticky.

Abdominal adhesions usually do not become noticed by doctors until they become very severe, but nonetheless may have a negative effect on many individuals recovering from chronic multisystem illness by impeding movement of waste through the intestinal tract.

When affecting the uterus, abdominal adhesions ("endometriosis") can interfere with fertility.

Helping the Intestinal Tract

Following are some measures that mold avoiders have reported to be helpful in addressing these diverse issues and increasing the functionality of the digestive tract.

* **Probiotics.** Good bacteria in the gut are said to dispose of at least 50 percent of the total toxic load acquired by healthy individuals. Reversing gut dysbiosis thus may be an effective detoxification tool. Homemade fermented foods (which contain many times more healthy bacteria than probiotic capsules) may be an effective way to do this. Paleo-oriented diets focused on improving the gut in "autoimmune" patients also may be helpful in decreasing dysbiosis. Prebiotics such as acacia fiber also may be helpful.

* **Cholestyramine.** Cholestyramine (CSM) is a binder that is particularly good at grabbing onto most biotoxins and carrying them out of the body in the stool. Some mold avoiders have found it to be an important part of their recovery. It is available only by prescription. Standard products contain artificial coloring plus either sugar or aspartame, but versions that are free of additives are available through compounding pharmacies. Some regular generic versions may be more tolerated than others. Although some mold illness patients have a very hard time taking this medication, it

tends to be tolerated much better when taken in a very good environment. Welchol is suggested by some doctors as an alternative.

* **Binders.** Although other substances may not be as good as CSM for removing biotoxins, they may be helpful in terms of removing the heavy metals or chemicals that usually also are problems for mold reactors. Some of these include brown seaweed, glucomannan, modified citrus pectin, chlorella, cilantro, activated charcoal, bentonite or other clays, apple pectin, arabinogalactan, acacia, oatmeal and potatoes.

* **Chelators.** These are especially helpful in binding to metals and carrying them out of the system, either through the urinary tract or the digestive tract. EDTA (available in IV, suppository, oral or soap formulas) is useful for lead and some other metals. For mercury, other chelators such as DMSA or ALA may be preferred. "Low and slow" may be the most effective chelation strategy for very ill individuals who are relatively early in the recovery process.

* **Laxatives.** Especially when binders are being used, keeping things moving out of the digestive tract may take some proactive effort. High doses of Vitamin C or magnesium may be especially appropriate since mold illness patients may benefit from these in other ways. Lactulose and aloe vera latex are said to exert an effect on the small intestine, which usually is a problem for individuals recovering from mold-related illness. Castor oil (used orally or rectally) also may be especially helpful in clearing the small intestine. Other kinds of herbal, over-the-counter or prescription laxatives may be appropriate as well.

* **Cleansing.** Colonics or enemas may be helpful in removing toxic materials from the intestines. Packaged preparations containing fiber and herbs (such as Perfect 7) also may be effective for this.

* **Enzymes.** Enzymes may be helpful in dissolving intestinal mucous or biofilms. They also may have benefits with regard to addressing intestinal adhesions. Abundant enzymes may be obtained in fresh produce juice. Enzymes also may be obtained in pill or capsule form (such as Wobenzym, pancreatin, nattokinase, serrapeptase, lumbrokinase). Okra Pepsin E3 is an enzyme-based product designed to dissolve mucous in the small intestine.

* **Marijuana.** Marijuana is an approved medical treatment for Crohn's disease in some states and may be helpful for other intestinal issues as well.

* **Supportive supplements.** Slippery elm, licorice and marshmallow are herbs that may help the gut, including the intestinal lining. Zinc and l-glutamine also may be helpful in helping with leaky gut, though the latter should be used with caution since it may be problematic for those with GABA/glutamate imbalances. Ginger is another herb thought to be very helpful for the gut.

* **Castor Oil Packs.** Castor oil packs may be helpful at drawing toxins out of the abdominal area.

* **Abdominal Massage.** Although abdominal massage is not routinely given by most massage therapists, insofar as adhesions are an issue it may be helpful. Self-care is also a possibility.

* **Ozone.** Ozone is a controversial treatment that, especially when used rectally, may have the potential of addressing intestinal adhesions and other gut problems.

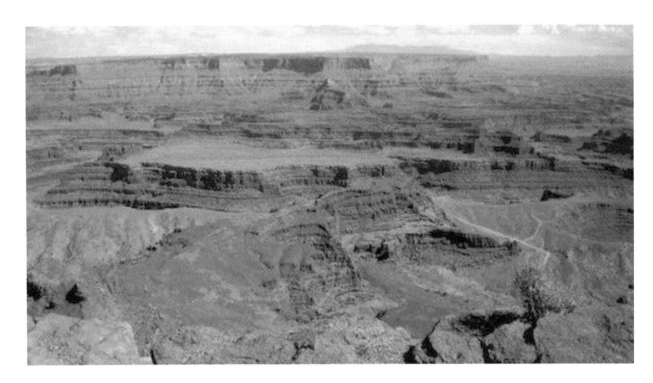

Dead Horse Point State Park near Moab, Utah.

Chapter 47

Detoxification: Sweating

Once toxins have been released from their storage places in the cells, an alternative way to remove them from the body may be by sweating them out.

Sweating thus may be especially helpful when other detoxification channels are impaired.

Like most other detoxification treatments, sweating tends to be much more effective in pristine locations than in more problematic ones.

Difficulties with Sweating

Especially when done in a more problematic place or early in recovery, promoting detoxification through sweating at a rapid rate can cause negative reactions.

Starting out slowly may be a good idea.

Individuals who are still very ill also may find that they have a difficult time sweating at all and thus should be careful when exposing themselves to heat.

Some mold avoiders have reported sweating out particularly problematic toxins with the potential of cross-contaminating clothing.

Washing off toxins excreted through sweat immediately may be helpful in preventing them from being reabsorbed into the body through the skin.

Spontaneous Sweating

Many individuals recovering from chronic multisystem disease experience spontaneous sweating episodes (which are similar to "hot flashes").

This seems to be an indicator that the body is overloaded with surface toxins that it is trying desperately to excrete.

Possibly it may be useful to consider these sweating episodes as indications that it could be worthwhile to detox in a more active way.

Because spontaneous sweating is hard on the system, the use of a sauna to produce sweat may be helpful for individuals experiencing sweating episodes.

Promoting Sweating

Following is a discussion of some different ways to help sweat be efficiently produced.

* **Exercise.** For those who are clear enough or well enough to exercise vigorously enough to sweat, this can be a good means of detoxification. Bikram or "hot" yoga may be especially effective at producing sweat at a moderate level of activity. Using water and a cloth to wipe off toxic sweat while exercising may be a good idea.

* **Infrared sauna.** This kind of sauna penetrates deep into the system and can be purchased for a relatively reasonable price for home use. Even a single infrared bulb in a lamp clamp has been reported as helpful in some cases.

* **Other treatments.** Regular saunas, steam rooms and hot springs baths all may be effective at encouraging the body to sweat. Regular baths at home (particularly Epsom salts baths) also may be helpful.

* **Hot weather.** Living without air conditioning in the summer can provide many of the benefits of a sauna, provided that it is possible to shower off the sweat and toxins on a regular basis. Many mold avoiders have stated that they believe that sweating in hot weather in a good environment (such as a clean desert) has been relatively pleasant and helpful to them.

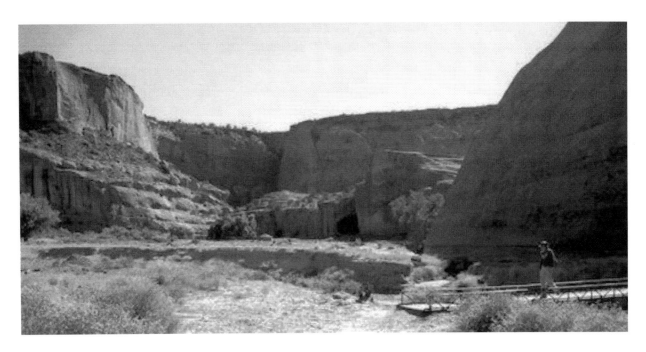

Canyon de Chelly National Monument near Chinle, Arizona.

Chapter 48

Food

Relatively few individuals with chronic multisystem disease tend to cite improved nutrition as having made a big difference in their health prior to pursuing mold avoidance.

Insofar as dietary changes have helped those individuals, it has tended to be as a result of avoiding problematic trigger foods rather than as a result of improving nutritional content.

However, many individuals with chronic multisystem conditions have stated that improved nutrition has made a huge difference for them once they started mold avoidance.

Detoxification and repair can be very be hard on the system, and supplying it with ample nutrients seems to make the process go more smoothly.

Many people have reported that their food reactivities have decreased after an extended period of mold avoidance, making a wider variety of foods available to them.

In the meantime, identifying and avoiding trigger foods is important in promoting optimal health gains.

Even after enough healing has occurred that food reactivities are not an issue, continuing to avoid both toxic contaminants of foods as well as "modern" foods that our bodies may not be adapted to handle easily may be a very good idea.

In general, a diet consisting only of fresh organic foods may be optimal.

This may not consist only of products labeled "organic" though, since many smaller producers grow or make foods without the use of chemicals but cannot afford to get the official certification.

Asking questions and relying on trustworthy growers is a good way to find out what has and hasn't been used.

Following is a discussion of some of the issues related to the consumption of various types of foods for individuals pursuing mold avoidance.

Produce

Incorporating as many colorful vegetables into the diet as possible may be helpful in providing the nutrients needed for the body to repair itself.

An optimal diet for those recovering from chronic multisystem illness might consist mostly of organic produce and high-quality fats, with other foods being minor players in comparison.

Although gut dysbiosis in particularly ill individuals may not allow them to tolerate sugars in fruits, mold avoiders who are farther along in the healing process may benefit from the enzymes and nutrients in them.

Similarly, juicing and green smoothies may be an efficient way of adding more vegetables and fruits to the diet for those individuals who are well enough to tolerate their sugar content.

Some mold avoiders have reported benefiting from up to 12 cups of fresh produce juice per day at points in their recovery process, for instance.

Although occasional juice fasts may be beneficial, whole raw and cooked produce generally are good to include as well since they provide different kinds of nutrients as well as fiber helpful in carrying out toxins.

217

The inclusion of ample amounts of fermented foods in the diet has been reported by some mold avoiders as having the potential of correcting some of their gut dysbiosis and thus allowing more sugars from produce to be tolerated.

Meat

Almost all supermarket and restaurant meat is quite toxic due to the practices used by industrial agriculture.

However, trichothecenes are protein synthesis inhibitors and animals (including humans) who have been negatively affected by these toxins may benefit from a diet that includes animal protein.

Including meats that have received only organic feed, GMO-free feed or grass in the diet – and preferably raised by small trustworthy farmers in places with good air quality - may be optimal.

Traditional cuts of meat - including such things as larger cuts on the bone and organ meats - may be particularly helpful.

Bone broth or chicken feet stock has been reported by some mold avoiders as being helpful as well.

Insofar as more conventional cuts of meat are the only choices available, the lean flesh tends to store fewer toxins than the fat and thus may be preferable.

Fats

Ample amounts of good-quality fats can be extremely helpful for those individuals recovering from toxic mold exposures.

The most beneficial fats may include organic olive oil (preferably from a small trusted California farmers since most products labeled "extra-virgin olive oil" actually contain other cheaper oils), organic coconut oil, organic avocado oil, and grass-fed or organic butter.

While a few individuals may have problems with the casein in butter, ghee appears to be tolerated by almost everyone.

Organic flaxseed oil or organic hempseed oil may be acceptable in relatively small quantities.

Organic walnut oil or other high-quality organic nut oils also may be considered acceptable fats.

Although mycotoxins and chemicals tend to be present in animal fat to a much higher degree than in animal flesh, bacon grease or lard from pigs fed very clean diets may be considered to be healthy fats.

"Modern" fats such as processed vegetable oils and margarine are harmful and should be avoided.

Fermented Foods

Homemade fermented foods contain many times more active good bacteria than probiotic supplements and can be very helpful for those attempting to heal the problems caused by gut dysbiosis.

Fermented foods that are fairly easy to make at home include milk kefir, yogurt, water kefir, kombucha, sauerkraut and other fermented vegetables, and condiments such as ketchup or mayonnaise.

While store-bought versions of these products often have few or no live cultures in them, certain brands of organic yogurt (such as Straus or Kalona Super Natural), organic sauerkraut (such as Farmhouse Cultures) or kombucha (such as GT's) do seem to have enough live cultures to make consumption worthwhile when homemade products are not available.

Some people have die-off reactions to incorporating large amounts of fermented foods into their diets.

In addition, those who are reactive to histamine can react negatively to some yogurts or certain other fermented foods.

Starting with a low amount of the particular food and carefully observing any negative reactions is suggested.

Vinegar

Natural vinegar (such as apple cider vinegar or balsamic vinegar) is a fermented food.

Although some brands may have chemical contamination issues, most mold avoiders seem to be fine with organic vinegar products.

Mushrooms

The fact that mushrooms are fungi tends to make many mold illness patients cautious about eating them.

However, mushrooms are non-toxic fungi and many experienced mold avoiders state that they have no problems eating mushrooms.

Some diets said to be particularly helpful for people with chronic multisystem illness (such as the Wahls Diet) advise that mushrooms be consumed on a regular basis.

Therapeutic mushrooms (such as chaga or reishi) may be helpful as well.

Fish and Seafood

Our oceans and other bodies of water are extremely contaminated with a variety of harmful substances, including heavy metals, chemicals, radiation and cyanotoxins.

Although fish and other seafood are inherently extraordinarily healthy foods, the contamination of the seafood currently available may have the potential of nullifying benefits, especially for those who already have an overabundance of toxicity in their systems.

For those who continue to eat seafood, choosing smaller non-farmed fish (such as salmon) may be a good idea.

Certain brands of sardines or other canned seafood (such as Wild Planet, Bela or Cole's) may be relatively low in toxicity as well.

Potatoes

Though potatoes are a traditional food that have been around in their current form for many years, some people with chronic multisystem disease report that they do better when they steer clear of them.

A few downsides of potatoes: the starch may have the ability to spike blood pressure or feed abnormal gut bacteria, and the anti-nutrients even in cooked potatoes may be difficult for people with gut dysbiosis to digest.

On the positive side, potatoes are a relatively inexpensive whole food that supply a reasonable amount of nutrients and may serve to effectively bind toxins in the gut.

For those who choose to eat potatoes, other types beside the standard russet (such as purple, yellow or red) may be preferred.

Nightshade Vegetables

Tomatoes, potatoes, peppers, eggplants and certain other foods have alkaloids that are difficult for some people with impaired gut function to digest.

Many mold avoiders find these otherwise healthy foods to be tolerable, however.

Dairy

A problem with dairy is that even if the cows obtain only organic feed and grass, mycotoxins from the feed are much more likely to make it into the milk than they are into lean animal flesh.

In addition, though it is risky for those with compromised immune systems to drink even the highest-quality raw milk, pasteurized milk is not an ideal food to be consuming either (in part because the good bacteria in raw milk helps to nullify toxins).

Other problems with dairy: many people with mold illness are reactive to casein, and milk sugars tend to promote the growth of intestinal worms.

Perhaps the best strategy with regard to fresh milk is to choose the best quality organic available and then to make it into homemade kefir or yogurt.

The fermentation will add good bacteria to the pasteurized milk and kill off any dangerous bacteria present in the raw milk.

It also will reduce the sugar content substantially.

For those who choose to eat cheese, purchasing cheese made in Europe rather than in the US may be worth considering since feed in Europe is more strictly regulated for mycotoxins and less likely to be contaminated with glyphosate.

Cheese made from cows that obtain mostly grass in their diets, such as Kerrygold, may be preferable.

High-fat dairy (such as whole milk or cream) seems preferable to reduced-fat for most purposes.

Industrial non-organic dairy products are extremely toxic and should be avoided.

Eggs

Eggs have the potential of being high in a variety of specific nutrients (such as choline and sulfur) that may be helpful to those recovering from mold illness.

However, eggs tend to be much more contaminated than meat by any mycotoxins or chemicals that the animal has ingested or inhaled.

If eggs are going to be consumed, then seeking out ones that are particularly high in quality (such as ones raised organically on pasture by small trustworthy farmers) may be worthwhile.

Even better could be to raise one's own chickens and feed them organic table scraps.

Commercial non-organic eggs are extremely toxic and should be avoided.

Nuts and Seeds

Nuts and seeds can be healthy foods, but unfortunately may be highly contaminated with mycotoxins even when grown organically.

Some organic nuts – such as almonds and pistachios – appear to be less likely to be contaminated with mold toxins than others.

Soaking nuts for even a few hours prior to using them may be helpful, since the mycotoxins as well as the natural anti-nutrients produced by the plant as a defense mechanism will be discarded with the soaking water.

Soaked nuts can be baked at a low temperature until they become crunchy again or can be made into homemade nut milks or nut butters.

Packaged nut butters are much more dicey, though some mold avoiders have very good things to say about some of the more expensive brands.

Legumes

Organic dried peas and beans contain natural anti-nutrients that may not be easy for individuals with gut dysbiosis to digest.

They also may be contaminated with mycotoxins.

Soaking these overnight prior to cooking and then discarding the soaking water can be helpful in addressing these problems.

Bottled Juices, Preserves and Dried Fruits

Even when the label says organic, processed or dried fruit products very often tend to be contaminated with problematic mycotoxins.

Soaking dried fruits before using may be somewhat helpful in removing these toxins.

Sticking with freshly made juices - which also contain more beneficial enzymes and nutrients - rather than consuming bottled ones is highly preferable.

High-quality purchased preserves may include less moldy fruit than lower-priced versions.

Wheat

Wheat has a number of characteristics that can make it problematic for those with chronic multisystem disease.

Commonly used wheat is a hybridized plant with a form of gluten that is much different than the one that was consumed by our ancestors.

This new form of gluten may be especially problematic for those with digestive tracts compromised by mold toxins.

In addition, even organic wheat is often contaminated with trichothecenes.

While some people are reactive enough to gluten that they likely will need to avoid all wheat permanently, others have found that some wheat products are much more tolerable for them than others.

For instance, Jovial (an Italian company) makes flour, pasta and cookies from organic Einkorn wheat - an ancient grain that may be more tolerated than modern wheat.

Some mold avoiders have found that organic wheat grown in Italy or other European countries (where mycotoxin standards are stricter than in the US) is relatively tolerable for them as well.

Other Grains

Many people who are recovering from chronic multisystem illness choose to minimize the amount of grains that they consume or eliminate grains wholly from the diet.

Most grains have the potential of being contaminated with mycotoxins and contain anti-nutrients that can be difficult for people with gut dysbiosis to digest.

Some grains, such as rice, can be highly contaminated with heavy metals as well.

Grains also tend to be much less nutritious than produce and to spike blood sugar.

Soaking grains such as rice, oats or quinoa prior to cooking may be helpful in reducing their toxicity content.

Insofar as grains are going to be consumed, choosing organic versions of more traditional forms (such as quinoa, rice or popcorn) from smaller trusted producers may be a good idea.

Soy

Organic soy products that are not fermented include estrogenic compounds that many people now believe to be problematic.

It may be best to keep consumption of these at a low level.

Fermented soy products such as soy sauce or miso apparently do not have this estrogenic issue and may be okay to consume if tolerated.

Conventional soy products that are not stated to be organic or GMO-free tend to be highly contaminated with glyphosate and should be avoided regardless of whether they are fermented.

Natural Sweeteners

Sugars of all kinds have the potential of worsening gut dysbiosis and feeding intestinal parasites.

They also are problematic for those with blood sugar stability issues.

For those who want small amounts of natural sweetening, raw honey (preferably produced by small growers in areas without commercial agriculture) or organic maple syrup may be acceptable choices.

Organic white sugar is good for feeding kombucha or water kefir grains but otherwise likely should be minimized even by those who can tolerate it.

Other Sweeteners

Stevia is obtained from a naturally sweet leaf of a South American plant.

However, most forms of it available in other places are highly processed, and many stevia products have added ingredients.

Xylitol is a heavily processed sweetener originating from wood pulp.

Using these sweeteners with caution, if at all, is suggested.

Although it is marketed as healthful, agave is a highly processed sugar.

Many people now believe agave is worse than refined cane sugar and should be avoided.

Artificial sweeteners originating from chemicals are toxic and should be carefully avoided.

Coffee and Cocoa

Both coffee and cocoa have the potential of being healthy foods, in part because they are high in antioxidants.

Dark chocolate has been found to be helpful for promoting the growth of healthy gut microorganisms as well.

However, both coffee and cocoa are often contaminated with ochratoxin.

Inexpensive brands seem to have more contamination than premium ones.

For those who are especially concerned, the organic products associated with the Bulletproof Executive are guaranteed to be low in mycotoxins.

Non-organic coffee can be highly contaminated with chemicals and likely should be avoided.

Although organic chocolate or cocoa is generally preferred, some non-organic products (especially those labeled as GMO-free) have been reported to be acceptable much of the time.

Teas and Spices

Both black and green tea have been shown in many research studies to have a positive effect in cases of mycotoxin poisoning.

Herbs and spices may have a variety of positive effects on the system.

Unfortunately, mycotoxin contamination is relatively common in many of these dried products.

Although it is possible that higher-quality brands will have less contamination, choosing to use fresh versions (such as garlic, ginger, parsley or basil) when available may be preferable.

Green tea may be less likely than black tea to be contaminated with mycotoxins.

Undenatured Whey Protein

Undenatured whey protein is said to have the ability to deliver usable glutathione to the liver, helping it to detoxify itself.

Depending on how the processing is done, it also may be high in colostrum (a substance that can help the immune system).

Grass-fed or organic products are strongly preferred.

Other whey protein is made from conventional dairy and likely should be avoided.

Supplements

The vast majority of vitamins and other dietary supplement products are made in China (a country with tremendous environmental toxicity problems) using very toxic processes.

Only a few companies (such as Pure Encapsulations) have their manufacturing facilities in the US or other countries.

Many other "natural" supplements contain mycotoxin contamination.

Although this does not mean that supplements will never be helpful, it does suggest that researching carefully how and where supplements are produced may be a good idea prior to using them.

When supplements seem important enough to be used despite the toxicity risks, choosing a quality brand may be a good idea.

Making an effort to obtain as much nutrition as possible from diet may be a better choice than relying on large quantities of supplements.

Alcohol

Ethanol is a mycotoxin, made by Saccharomyces yeast.

In general, most humans' livers are able to detoxify this type of mycotoxin relatively easily.

However, a number of studies have shown that the combination of ethanol with other mycotoxins results in much more damage than if the ethanol were not present.

In addition, many types of alcohol tend to be very contaminated with dangerous mycotoxins, and these are not removed in the distilling process.

Wines (especially those made in the US) and lower-quality products may be especially likely to be contaminated with mycotoxins as well as other toxic contaminants.

In general, caution with regard to alcohol is advisable for those with mold illness.

When alcohol is consumed, sticking with products made in Europe (which has comparably good standards with regard to mycotoxin levels) or high-quality brands may be a good idea.

Canned and Frozen Produce

While organic canned or frozen foods tend to have less nutrition than fresh food, they may be options when fresh food is not available.

A main problem with canned food is that the can liners almost invariably contain BPA or similar chemicals.

Glass containers (especially for acidic foods like tomatoes) may be safer.

Some organic frozen produce originates from China, so checking the labels may be a good idea.

Processed and Restaurant Foods

In general, avoiding both processed foods and restaurant foods as much as possible is something to consider.

Although these are convenient, they usually are laden with a variety of toxins, problematic fats and poor-quality ingredients.

Processed organic foods are somewhat preferable to processed non-organic foods, but still do not have the health-giving benefits of homemade foods prepared with quality ingredients.

At restaurants that do not promise organic food, sticking with salads and steamed vegetables (preferably bringing dressing or butter from home) may be safer than consuming other items on the menu.

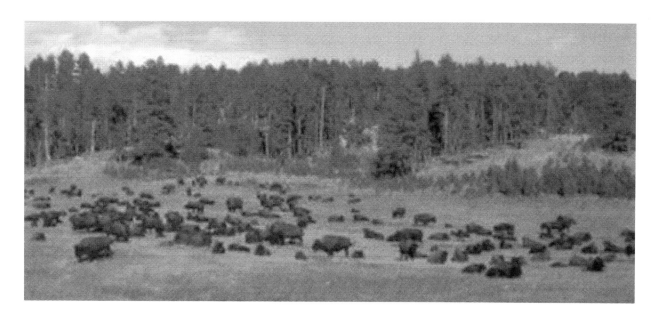

Buffalo grazing near Wind Cave National Park in South Dakota.

Chapter 49

Pathogens

People suffering from chronic multisystem disease invariably are infected with a wide variety of pathogens.

A few of the pathogens commonly seen in patients with chronic multisystem disease include herpes family viruses of all kinds (including HHV6, EBV, CMV, HSV, herpes zoster), enteroviruses, borrelia (commonly known as Lyme), systemic bacteria (such as bartonella, chlamydophila pneumoniae or coxiella burnetii), fungi (such as aspergillus, coccidioides or candida), mycoplasma, systemic parasites (such as babesia, ehrlichia or toxoplasma), intestinal protozoa (such as cryptosporidium), and multi-celled parasites (such as tapeworms, hookworms or liver flukes).

The fact that none of these pathogens seems to be present in all patients and that all pathogens tend to be very resistant to treatments that work well in people without this type of disease and in the laboratory suggests that underlying immune system deficits may be reasonably viewed as the cause of their presence.

One possibility is that toxins stored in the system are responsible for these immune system issues.

More than 200 peer-reviewed papers in the medical literature discuss the ability of trichothecenes to cause many different kinds of immune system problems.

Chemicals and heavy metals may have the potential to contribute to the ability of pathogens to establish themselves in the system as well.

While it may be that a high percentage of the harm done by trichothecenes to the system is via the various pathogens that establish themselves, that does not necessarily mean that directly attacking the pathogens is the most effective course of action.

Although treating the pathogens may result in immediate health gains in individuals at a moderate level of toxicity, those gains very well may dissipate over time unless the underlying toxicity issue is addressed.

For individuals at a higher level of toxicity, no specific treatments may be sufficient to get the pathogens under control.

Die-off symptoms tend to be severe in this population, often with little noticeable subsequent improvement in the problem.

For the most part, treating pathogens of all kinds is much easier and more effective for people when they are in a good environment rather than in a more problematic one.

Successful detoxification of the system may have the potential of making treatment of pathogens more successful as well, in terms of both the ease of treating the infection as well as the likelihood that it will remain under control instead of re-emerging later on.

Toxin-Producing Microorganisms

Some pathogens appear to produce toxins that are particularly detrimental to patients with chronic multisystem disease.

Borrelia, certain fungal infections and intestinal worms frequently have been suggested as being able to make damaging toxins, but other infections also may have this ability.

An often considered question is whether it is better to focus first on the toxin component of the illness (such as through avoidance and detoxification) or on the pathogen component.

In general, if an individual is tolerating a pathogen treatment fairly easily (without experiencing a substantial Herxheimer response), then continuing that treatment if it seems valuable may be a reasonable thing to do.

On the other hand, if a particular treatment is prompting a difficult die-off, then the experiences of many mold avoiders suggest that it may be worth considering postponing that treatment until after getting to a better environment and possibly until after engaging in some detoxification.

Very commonly, infections may be much easier to treat - or may resolve spontaneously so that they do not need to be treated - after the toxic component of the illness is addressed.

Viruses

Due at least in part to the low natural killer cell activity common in this sort of disease, herpes family viruses often reactivate and cause large amounts of inflammation that may exacerbate mold reactivity. Following are some commonly used treatments.

* **Antiviral drugs.** Valcyte, Famvir and Valtrex have been reported by a few mold avoiders as somewhat helpful at decreasing mold reactivity, improving cognition and addressing certain other symptoms. However, these drugs have been known to make some patients (especially those living in problematic environments) substantially worse, and some who take the drugs do not return to baseline after stopping them. Considering environmental factors before pursuing these drugs may be a good idea.

* **Olive leaf extract.** This is an herb that may have positive effects on the immune system in general, particularly with regard to killing viruses. It tends to diminish in effectiveness when taken on a continuous basis.

* **Ozone.** Although controversial, ozone is said to have the ability to address all kinds of pathogens including viruses.

Fungi

Pathogenic fungi of all kinds may be issues for those with chronic multisystem disease.

Illnesses caused may include coccidioidomycosis ("Valley Fever"), cryptococcus, aspergillosis, histoplasmosis, candidiasis and others.

It is possible that these fungi produce toxins inside the body, causing similar effects to what people would experience if they were breathing in mycotoxins.

In cases where the immune system is suppressed, candida in the intestinal system has the ability to extend into other parts of the body.

Candida therefore may have more far-reaching negative effects than most people realize.

For instance, candida pushing on the inner ear (or growing into it) may cause severely life-limiting vertigo.

Other kinds of fungal infections can be even more problematic.

A particular problem with regard to treatment is that fungi tend to become resistant to medications as well as supplements very quickly.

Therefore, even if a medication provides quick relief, it cannot be counted upon to be a solution into the future.

A possible underlying cause of all these fungal infections is that trichothecenes (including those being breathed in from current exposures as well as those sequestered in the system from previous exposures) are having a negative effect on the immune system, making people more susceptible to other pathogenic fungi.

If that is the case, then continued avoidance and detoxification may be more effective at successfully controlling these pathogens over the long term than any medication or other treatment.

For the short term though, here are some treatment alternatives.

Die-off reactions may be strong with all of these, so proceeding slowly may be a good idea.

* **Diet.** A diet that is as low as possible in sugars and starches will give candida and perhaps some other fungi less fuel to grow on. An exception may be carrot juice, which is high in natural sugars but may be helpful in controlling candida.

* **Natural treatments.** A variety of supplements may be helpful in controlling fungal infections throughout the system. These may include berberines (such as goldenseal), garlic, pau d'arco, coconut oil (and its derivative caprylic acid), grapefruit seed extract, oregano oil and certain kinds of enzymes. Rotating these may be advisable.

* **Sinus treatments.** Sinus infections are common in chronic multisystem disease, and most sinus infections are caused by fungi. A combination of an anti-fungal drug (such as amphotericin B) and an anti-biofilm agent (such as EDTA) is often incorporated in nasal spray or cream. A few mold avoiders have said good things about Super Good Stuff Nasal Wash, a natural product. Rinsing the sinuses periodically with a Neti pot also may be helpful. (Note that only distilled or boiled water should be used in Neti pot since dangerous infections otherwise can result. The addition of Johnson's Baby Shampoo sometimes has been suggested as a way to break up biofilms.)

* **Nystatin.** This is a drug that stays within the intestinal tract and that may be helpful in controlling candida there.

* **Systemic antifungal drugs.** Drugs such as fluconazole may be effective in controlling systemic fungal infections in the short term, but it is best not to count on them since resistance usually emerges with long-term use.

* **Ozone.** Though controversial, ozone may have the potential of controlling fungi in the intestinal tract and elsewhere without the problem of resistance seen when drugs are used.

* **Detox.** Keeping things moving in the digestive tract is especially important when killing intestinal fungi, since otherwise the toxins released can produce huge die-off reactions. Colonics, enemas or laxatives may be helpful for this.

Bacteria & Mycoplasma

Borrelia (commonly known as Lyme) is a bacteria that appears to have the ability to create toxins that cause symptoms similar to those of mold toxins.

Some people believe that certain genetically susceptible individuals have a difficult time eliminating these toxins from their systems, thus causing or contributing to the development of chronic multisystem disease.

Other systemic bacteria and mycoplasma may produce inflammatory toxins as well.

Individuals who already have chronic multisystem disease tend to be especially susceptible to these pathogens, meaning that they may have a hard time getting them under control even with antibiotics.

Pathogenic gut bacteria also are common in this sort of disease.

Some of these gut bacteria may be particularly problematic because they produce LPS, a substance that acts synergistically with trichothecenes to cause particularly deleterious effects.

Bacteria with the potential of causing food poisoning (such as campylobacter or salmonella) may present a particularly great threat to those who already are ill with chronic multisystem disease.

Antibiotic-resistant bacteria may be especially life-threatening to individuals who have had their immune systems compromised as a result of this kind of disease.

As with other pathogens, decreasing environmental stress on the system through mold avoidance may be helpful in getting all of these infections under control.

Here are some additional treatments reported to be helpful.

* **Detoxification.** The importance of actively pursuing detoxification while treating borrelia and related pathogens is widely recognized in the Lyme community, since patients otherwise tend to get very sick from the toxins released as the microorganisms die off. Detoxification also may make the immune system stronger, thus allowing infections to be brought under control more easily (in some cases without any treatment at all).

* **Antibiotics.** While the short-term use of antibiotics for bacterial and mycoplasma infections is widely accepted as appropriate, longer-term use of these drugs is a much more controversial choice. While some individuals with chronic multisystem disease state that they feel better as a result of being on the drugs for extended periods of time, antibiotics have a number of negative characteristics: they are destructive of the good bacteria in the gut; they may prompt unpleasant die-off reactions; and they have the propensity to make infections more resistant by prompting the formation of biofilms. Antibiotics have been reported by many mold avoiders to work much better with less die-off in good environments than in problematic ones.

* **Herbs.** A wide variety of herbs and other nutritional supplements have been reported to be effective in treating borrelia and other bacterial infections. One advantage of herbs over prescription antibiotics is that they usually do not seem to have a negative effect on the good bacteria of the system. Still, they can prompt substantial die-off reactions. In addition, if the system remains overly toxic, the pathogens that have been killed may be very likely to return. Again, many mold avoiders report that these are easier to take and more effective in better environments.

* **Probiotics.** Increasing the amount of good bacteria in the gut via fermented foods or supplements may help to crowd out pathogens and also improve the immune system.

* **Hyperbaric oxygen therapy (HBOT).** Problematic bacteria generally tend to thrive in low-oxygen environments such as those of the systems of many individuals with chronic multisystem disease. Periodically forcing oxygen into the tissues of the system may help to control infections. Some medical practitioners offer treatments to patients for a fee. HBOT chambers also may be rented or purchased for home use.

* **Ozone.** While controversial, ozone has been reported by many individuals with chronic multisystem disease (including some of those pursuing mold avoidance) as helpful for borrelia and a variety of other pathogens. While the initial investment may be expensive (often $600-1500), the equipment can be used repeatedly and tends to have good resale

value. Trying out ozone in the office of a health care practitioner or with a water ozonator before purchasing expensive equipment may be a good idea.

* **Vitamin C IV's.** At higher doses, these have the ability to kill pathogens such as borrelia and other bacteria. The mechanism is that any Vitamin C that the system cannot immediately use turns into H202 (hydrogen peroxide).

* **Sinus treatments.** MARCoNS is an antibiotic resistant bacteria that some mold illness doctors report often finding in the sinuses of patients with mold illness. BEG nasal spray (suggested by Dr. Ritchie Shoemaker) includes a combination of antibiotics as well as EDTA chelation to break up biofilms. Natural sinus treatments may also be effective.

Intestinal Parasites

Multi-celled parasites such as tapeworms, hookworms and liver flukes have been increasingly recognized in recent years as a previously underestimated problem for many individuals with chronic multisystem illness.

Most of these organisms are toxin producers.

Some intestinal parasites (particularly tapeworms) also can consume enormous quantities of B vitamins (especially B12) as well as other nutrients.

Their presence in the system appears to be related to the potential for reactivation of herpes family viruses.

An important issue for people with chronic multisystem disease is that worms are capable of sequestering enormous amounts of heavy metals (and perhaps other poisons as well) in their systems.

Possibly they are using this as a defense against the immune system.

Killing the worms too rapidly has the potential of releasing these heavy metals into the system, causing it severe harm.

Even mold avoiders who have felt quite well for a long time may have the potential of being negatively affected by the release of these heavy metals.

Therefore, intestinal parasites (especially in people who have been showing symptoms for many years) need to be approached with great care.

While it may be that true health never will be obtained while these parasites remain in the system, being too aggressive in attempting to kill them may possibly be a mistake.

Following are some treatments that are often discussed with regard to multi-celled intestinal parasites.

* **Biofilm removers.** Intestinal parasites tend to be covered with biofilms, making them relatively resistant to treatments designed to kill them. The biofilms also often have a heavy metal component incorporated in them. Some biofilm removers include various kinds of enzymes (such as lumbrokinase, serrapeptase, nattokinase, pepsin, Wobenzym or large amounts of fresh juice), monolaurin (a component of coconut oil), cloves, or EDTA.

* **Removal of heavy metals.** As worms die off, heavy metals are released into the system. Measures that help to remove these metals may prevent the individual from becoming much more ill and also allow the parasites to be killed more effectively without the ability to reestablish themselves later on. Some potential tools for removing metals from the system include sweating (such as through infrared sauna or exercise); EDTA or other chelators; brown seaweed; optimizing methylation; binders; juicing; coffee enemas; and increasing good bacteria in the intestines through fermented foods.

* **Fasting.** Worms absorb semi-digested food as it moves through their host's intestines and may tolerate a lack of food less well than their human hosts. A water fast or a fresh juice fast may be helpful. Worms especially tend to like sugar and dairy products, and so eliminating just these from the diet may be helpful for weakening parasites.

* **Produce.** Worms are much less likely to thrive when a vegan diet is consumed even for a discrete period of time. Despite being high in sugar, carrot juice and some other juices have been reported as highly effective at addressing intestinal worms.

* **Herbs.** Herbal combinations designed to address intestinal parasites tend to include artemesia, clove, black walnut hulls, garlic and pumpkin seeds. Certain Traditional Chinese Medicine (TCM) herbs may be effective as well. Herbs tend to work gradually on parasites which, considering the heavy metals issue, could be a good thing.

* **Diatomaceous earth.** This is a powdery substance that contains tiny sharp shards of diatoms (microorganisms similar to cyanobacteria). These have the ability to cut through the skin of worms, making them more inclined to dry out and die. In theory this is said not to harm humans or other mammals when taken internally, although it has been questioned whether (especially for people with leaky gut) it is really a good idea to consume it. Using it for limited periods of time, if at all, may be best.

* **Salt/C Protocol.** Salt may have the ability to dehydrate and kill worms, and the addition of Vitamin C is said to have the ability of making this treatment more effective.

* **Ozone.** Ozone therapy is a controversial treatment that may have the ability to kill pathogens throughout the body. Intestinal parasites may be included in this, especially when the ozone is used rectally.

* **Drugs.** A variety of drugs (including praziquantel, pyrantel pamoate and ivermectin) are said to have the ability to kill intestinal parasites. These often work less well in those with chronic multisystem disease than they do in other populations, perhaps due to the presence of larger amounts of metals, more established biofilms or weaker overall immune systems. Many patients have reported getting worse as a result of taking these drugs, in some cases for a long time. Caution is advised.

* **Chlorine dioxide.** Of all the treatments mentioned in this book, this may be the most controversial. However, a number of people with chronic multisystem illness (including a few mold avoiders) have reported effectively killing parasites and making health gains specifically from using this substance.

Systemic Parasites

Systemic parasites can be amongst the most damaging pathogens in existence.

Those with chronic multisystem disease may be especially susceptible to them.

Babesiosis and toxoplasmosis tend to be fairly frequently reported in this patient population, for instance.

Systemic parasites tend to be very difficult to kill with available drugs or herbs in this patient population.

Drugs tend to be toxic, die-off reactions tend to be fierce, and even when improvements do occur the parasites tend to resurface when treatments are stopped.

However, these parasites usually become an issue only when the immune system is very severely compromised.

Improving immune system function even somewhat may prompt substantial improvement or resolution of symptoms generated by these pathogens.

Therefore, it may be that taking measures to improve the immune system functioning (such as with mold avoidance, detoxification and gut repair) may be a worth considering before pursuing aggressive treatment of these infections with drugs or herbs.

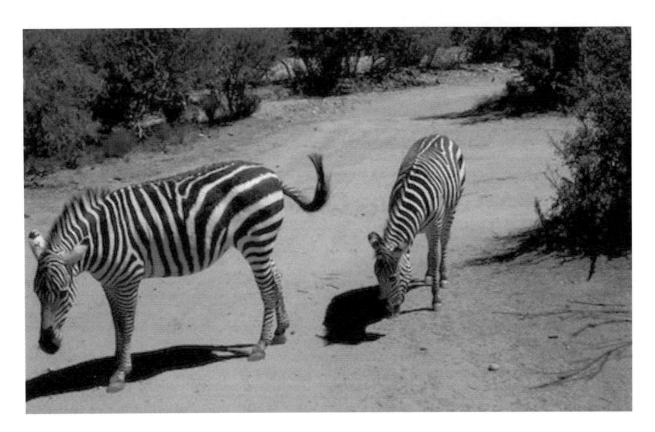

Zebras at the ethical wildlife park Out of Africa in Camp Verde, Arizona.

Chapter 50

Medical Care

Many individuals with chronic multisystem disease have reported that treatments of all kinds tend to be much more effective when pursued in combination with mold avoidance.

Working with a physician or other practitioner knowledgeable about this type of illness is necessary to obtain some kinds of testing or treatments and also may be helpful in developing an effective treatment plan and predicting the likely effects that particular treatments are likely to produce.

Knowledgeable physicians may include mold illness specialists; functional or integrative medical practitioners; ME/CFS specialists; and Lyme literate medical doctors.

Many of these physicians will work with patients via telephone, especially after the initial consultation.

Following are some tests and treatments that have been reported as helpful by some mold avoiders and that require a relationship with a practitioner to obtain.

Testing

* **Mold illness markers.** Many physicians focusing on mold illness use the series of tests developed by Dr. Ritchie Shoemaker to diagnose the condition and to gauge how well individuals are doing as they attempt to return to health through avoidance and treatment. Included are the following laboratory tests: MSH, TGF beta-1, C4a, AGA (antigliadin antibodies), ACTH/cortisol, VEGF, ACLA (anticardiolipin antibodies), ADH/Osmolality, MMP9, and Leptin.

* **Mold illness susceptibility.** Shoemaker also suggests looking at HLA DR to determine the extent to which individuals have the propensity to become ill from exposures to mycotoxins. He states that about 25% of the population is susceptible to becoming ill from mold toxicity and that about 2% of the population has the propensity to become ill with ME/CFS or similar conditions.

* **Mycotoxin tests.** RealTime Laboratories offers a test that measures the amount of three different kind of mycotoxins (aflatoxin, ochratoxin and trichothecene) in the urine. The presence of at least one of these mycotoxins was reported in one paper to be very common (almost ubiquitous) in patients with ME/CFS or related conditions.

* **Mold allergy tests.** IgG tests provide information on the extent to which individuals recently have been exposed to a variety of different molds (including Stachybotrys). They thus can be viewed as an alternative to environmental testing in determining whether individuals have recently been living or working in a problematic environment. IgE tests measure commonplace allergies to common molds (toxic and non-toxic) and are of little help in providing information about the extent to which people are being affected by mold toxicity.

* **ME/CFS tests.** Doctors specializing in the condition called ME/CFS (which they may or may not associate with mold illness) have found a number of abnormalities that are typical of their patient base. These include low natural killer cell function, low suppressor T-cells (and low suppressor/helper T-cell ratios), Type 1 diastolic dysfunction, reactivated herpes family viruses (such as EBV, CMV or HHV6), elevated apoptosis levels and Rnase-L fragmentation. Improvements in these measures may suggest healing progress.

* **Methylation pathway tests.** This test provides information on the functioning of the methylation system, which tends to be a particular problem in ME/CFS sufferers as well as many others with chronic multisystem disease. The test includes information on the status of glutathione (reduced and oxidized), S-adenosyl-methionine, S-adenosyl-

homocysteine, tetrahydrofolate, 5-methyl-THF, 10-formyl-THF, 5-formyl-THF, folic acid, folinic acid and adenosine.

* **Methylation and detox genetic tests.** 23andMe provides a list of genetics to individuals based on a saliva sample. Then a program such as Genetic Genie can be used to find out what these polymorphisms mean in terms of likely health effects. Although a physician is not needed for either of these, certain medical practitioners may be helpful in providing information on how to address particular detoxification issues.

In-Office Treatments

Following is a list of treatments administered in physicians' offices that some individuals pursuing mold avoidance have found to be helpful.

* **Nutritional IV's.** Vitamin C IV's are helpful at decreasing oxidative stress, promoting detoxification and killing pathogens. Other IV's that have been reported as being helpful include ALA, glutathione, B12, other B vitamins, magnesium, zinc, and other minerals. For those experiencing orthostatic intolerance, the saline solution infusion from the IV may be helpful as well.

* **Chelation.** Chelation agents such as EDTA or DMSA bind with heavy metals in the system, allowing those metals to be removed. Although this sounds like a good idea, loosening up metals in an aggressive way can cause patients at a higher level of toxicity to feel much worse. However, for those patients who can tolerate it, this can be an effective means of systemic detoxification.

* **Hyperbaric oxygen therapy (HBOT).** HBOT has been reported by some mold avoiders of having the potential of promoting wound healing, pathogen killing and improved cognitive functioning. Some doctors have a small chamber in their own offices; others may write a prescription for treatment to be obtained at a specialty center.

* **Neural therapy.** This technique involves injecting small amounts of various substances (such as procaine, homeopathic remedies or vitamins) into trigger points, scars or other sensitive areas of the body. It can be helpful in facilitating detoxification and relieving pain for those with drainage issues.

* **Ampligen.** This is an experimental drug available by IV only from certain doctors specializing in ME/CFS. It may be effective at helping with a variety of symptoms related to chronic multisystem illness, but the cost can be as high as $50,000 per year out-of-pocket.

* **Intravenous immunoglobulin (IVIG).** This is a blood product from the pooled plasma of more than a thousand donors, designed to help to improve antibody function in immunocompromised patients. It is another expensive treatment offered by only a few doctors.

General Medications

Following are some prescription medications that mold avoiders have found to be helpful for them during their healing process.

* **Cholestyramine (CSM).** This powdered medication binds with toxins in the intestines and carries them out of the body in the stool. It is thought to have a particular propensity to bind to mold toxins. CSM is available with sugar and artificial coloring through regular pharmacies or without additives through compounding pharmacies. Welchol is a prescription alternative.

* **Vasoactive intestinal peptide (VIP).** This is a treatment first proposed by Dr. Ritchie Shoemaker for mold illness patients, based on the idea that certain regulatory neuropeptides (MSH and VIP) tend to be insufficiently high in this population. Although Shoemaker recommends it only for individuals who are pursuing avoidance to a sufficient extent to have recovered some of their health, ME/CFS physician Dr. Paul Cheney suggests that he believes it may be helpful for his patients (especially with regard to promoting normal liver flow) as well. VIP is available in a nasal spray through certain compounding pharmacies.

* **B12 shots.** Especially at certain points during recovery, some patients benefit from very large amounts of B12, such as can be delivered only through injections. Hydroxycobalmin or methylcobalmin tend to be preferred.

* **Deplin.** Deplin is a prescription medication (dubbed a "medical food") providing in pill form large amounts of methyl folate, the activated form of the B vitamin folic acid. This particular substance often is deficient in those with methylation issues, and some patients have reported benefiting from large amounts of it at certain points during their recovery processes. Lower amounts of methyl folate are available in supplements available without a prescription.

* **Low-dose naltrexone (LDN).** LDN appears to serve as a modulator for the immune system, in some cases allowing it to do a better job of killing pathogens and reacting to other threats. A few mold avoiders have reported finding it to be helpful.

* **Bioidentical hormone replacement.** Even after considerable avoidance, many individuals with chronic multisystem illness have a variety of hormone levels that are lower than would be expected in people who are not ill. These may include DHEA,

progesterone, testosterone, certain forms of estrogen, cortisol, T3 and growth hormone. While there is not universal agreement that this always is a good idea, some patients have reported improvements as a result of supplementing bioidentical versions of these hormones so that more normal levels are achieved.

* **Benzodiazapines.** Klonopin and other benzodiazapines are tranquilizers that are often used to protect the brains of sea otters and other mammals from the negative effects of aquatic biotoxins such as domoic acid. Some ME/CFS doctors have observed a protective effect in humans with chronic multisystem disease as well, suggesting that the drugs can temporarily address GABA/glutamate imbalances and promote improved sleep. Although those successfully pursuing mold avoidance often report these drugs to be unnecessary for them to get good sleep, they may be helpful for those who have yet to get wholly clear. The amino acid L-theanine may be an option.

* **Anticonvulsants.** Mold illness patients often have issues related to seizures or convulsions, including mood swings. Lamictal or other anticonvulsants may be helpful for this.

* **Florinef.** This drug can help to counter the orthostatic intolerance that many chronic multisystem disease patients experience prior to or early in the recovery process.

* **Beta blockers.** Beta blockers are commonly used in ME/CFS for treatment of POTS, a type of orthostatic intolerance. Anecdotally, POTS tends to be related to exposure to the Mystery Toxin and generally fades with successful avoidance of that toxic substance. However, for those who are experiencing POTS symptoms, beta blockers may be helpful.

* **Laxatives.** Trichothecenes tend to have a negative effect on the small intestine, with blockages often resulting. Certain medications such as lactulose sometimes may have a positive effect when other approaches fail.

* **Medical marijuana.** An increasing number of states offer this as an option. Some patients find it helpful for pathogen killing, pain, sleep, nausea, cognition, infections, intestinal dysfunction or emotional issues. It also may have anticonvulsant properties. Cannabis oil is thought by some to be more effective than smoking the plant.

* **Immune suppressants.** Some doctors view ME/CFS and other similar chronic multisystem illnesses as "autoimmune" conditions. This term suggests that they believe that the system is reacting in a mistaken way against itself or against benign environmental triggers. Thus, they suggest certain medications (such as adalimumab, infliximab, etanercept or rituximab) that selectively turn off certain parts of the immune system. Although this sort of approach occasionally has been reported as having had impressive short-term effects, apparent longer-term consequences have in some cases been strongly negative (with individuals falling into a deeper level of illness). Insofar as

the immune system is reacting appropriately against an actual threat that would do it harm (such as particular biotoxins that it is already overloaded with), turning off the immune system's response would logically be expected to cause negative effects over the long-term. Approaching these kinds of drugs with extreme caution therefore may be a good idea for this patient population.

Anti-Pathogen Medications

* **Viruses.** Many individuals with ME/CFS (including many of those successfully pursuing mold avoidance) have chronic issues with herpes family viruses, due at least in part to low natural killer cell function. A few mold avoiders have noted that use of antiviral drugs (such as Valtrex, Famvir or Valcyte) has decreased their mold reactivity a bit, improved their cognition and had other positive effects.

* **Intestinal parasites.** Increasing attention has become focused on the tendency of patients with chronic multisystem illness to acquire a wide variety of worms and flukes. Drugs such as praziquantel, pyrantel pamoate or ivermectin may be prescribed to treat the problem, though (as discussed in Chapter 49) these should be used with extreme care.

* **Fungi.** Although fungi tend to become resistant to medications quickly, using antifungal drugs to get them under control in the short-term can be useful in some cases. This could include systemic drugs such as Diflucan. Treatment of sinus fungi (using a combination of amphotericin B and chelators designed to dissolve protective biotoxins) also has been used by some physicians.

* **Bacteria and mycoplasma.** Especially for patients at a lower level of systemic toxicity, antibiotics (such as doxycyline or azithromycin) may be effective at getting infections under control. Decreased mold reactivity sometimes has been reported. A downside of antibiotic use involves the possibility of long-term negative effects on gut bacteria as well as increased formation of biofilms in the gut.

* **Systemic parasites.** Protozoa cause certain systemic diseases such as toxoplasmosis or babesiosis. Since generally these diseases emerge only when the immune system is very weak, mold avoidance and related treatments often may be more effective at addressing the problem than pharmaceutical options. However, drug treatments may be available.

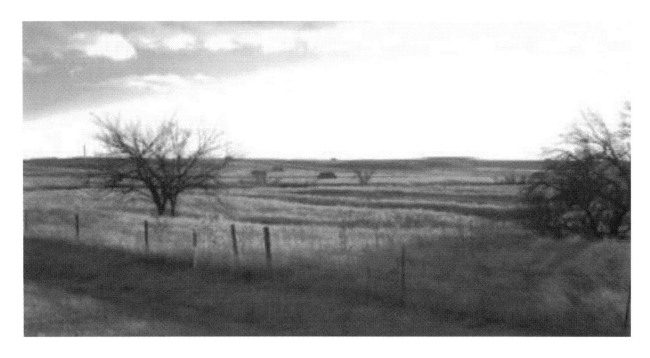

Near Sidney, Nebraska.

Chapter 51

Emotional Recovery

Most mold avoiders state that they believe that their illness was primarily driven by physiological factors.

However, considering the role that neurotoxins play in chronic multisystem illnesses, it is not surprising that emotional issues can play a role during the recovery process.

Regaining Emotional Fulfillment

Being ill with chronic multisystem illness is almost always extremely taxing at an emotional and spiritual level.

As a direct result of the neurotoxins exposures, individuals often feel that they have either become emotionally numb or that their emotions have lost all relationship to what is actually going on in their lives.

Reclaiming a positive life at a spiritual level after having been sick for an extended amount of time and within the constraints of avoidance may be a challenge.

Recovering a sense of having a rich and rewarding emotional and spiritual life can take time.

In addition, mold avoidance can be a tremendously difficult endeavor requiring a great deal of commitment and determination.

Almost without exception, people who have pursued it successfully have had a particular purpose in mind with regard to why it has been worth it to them.

In some cases this has been related to other people, such as wanting to be able to take care of a child or be in a relationship.

In others it has been with regard to missing part of the self that has been lost, such as the desire to regain the ability to do intellectual work or to exercise.

Many of those individuals who have recovered at least some of their health through mold avoidance have been drawn to making efforts to help other illness sufferers.

Considering in advance and then keeping in mind the reasons for wanting to pursue this endeavor may be helpful in making it seem more worthwhile on a day-to-day basis.

Finding ways to have fun and to socialize with others while pursuing mold avoidance is something that often takes effort but nonetheless may be worthwhile.

Brain Retraining

One technique that is often discussed in the environmental illness community is that of amygdala or brain retraining.

This is designed to encourage the system to stop hyperreacting to certain environmental stimuli.

For the most part, brain retraining seems based on the hypothesis that people are reacting inappropriately to stimuli that should not be harmful to them.

Brain retraining has some success stories amongst patients with reactivities to things like fabrics, wood smoke or mild chemicals.

However, thus far we have received no reports of mold avoiders finding it to be instrumental in addressing their own mold reactivities.

Possibly relevant is the fact that the known effects of certain biotoxins may have the ability to create the conditions under which people may become hyperreactive to many other substances.

Stachybotrys is able to create perforations in the blood-brain barrier, and certain aquatic biotoxins with symptoms similar to those of the Mystery Toxin are known to have a destabilizing and kindling effect on the hippocampus and amygdala if they are able to get into the brain.

The combination of these two toxins may have the ability to create a scenario where the brain becomes destabilized enough that reactivities to a wide variety of substances may occur.

In any event, the principle of mold avoidance is based on the idea of becoming very good at identifying particularly harmful environmental toxins and thus controlling exposures to them.

Insofar as small amounts of particular substances are actually causing harm (rather than acting as mere autoimmune triggers), then it likely would be inappropriate to turn off warning symptoms to exposures to them with brain retraining or drugs.

On the other hand, in a few instances experienced mold avoiders have reported that even after large amounts of detoxification and substantial decreases in terms of being negatively affected by exposures to particular toxins, their ability to sense particular mold toxins in the environment remained very high.

At that point, making a purposeful decision not to become upset by the identification of tiny amounts of cross-contamination in the environment was helpful in moving toward a more normal life.

In general, an ideal of mold avoidance is to be able to sense the presence of toxins in the environment and then to make a considered decision about how to handle them based on their expected negative effects.

Although it may be easier said than done, looking at warning symptoms as information rather than as behavioral mandates may allow some mold avoiders to feel less stressed and more in control.

Finally, it is possible that brain retraining might be helpful for individuals who are reacting to the proteins in non-toxic mold spores rather than to the mold toxins.

Actual instances of mold avoiders being helped by this have yet to be reported to us, however.

Part 6

CONSTRUCTION, TESTING & REMEDIATION

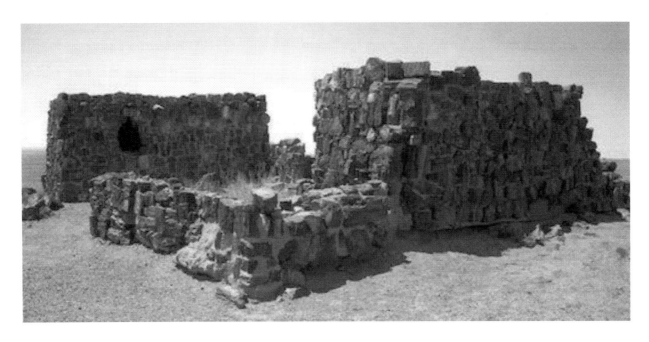

Agate House at Petrified National Forest near Holbrook, Arizona.

Chapter 52

Mold-Resistant Construction

Very often when new mold avoiders realize that they are having a difficult time tolerating most or all conventional housing, they consider the possibility of building a dwelling that would be guaranteed as safe for them.

Generally this turns out to be a remarkably difficult undertaking.

Building a house that will remain mold-free enough to be safe for healthy people is a comparatively simple proposition, provided that most conventional building techniques (such as drywall, wall insulation and HVAC systems) are eliminated.

Creating a residence that will for sure be livable into the future for someone who has become an extreme reactor to toxic mold is much more challenging.

As a result, although many mold avoiders have considered the possibility of building their own mold-safe homes, thus far very few have gone forward with this sort of project.

For those who are interested in the idea of pursuing it, here are some thoughts.

Potential Pitfalls

Those considering building or buying a mold-safe residence may do well to think carefully about all the things that could prevent them either from finishing the project or from living in it successfully over the long term.

One risk in investing in any non-movable home is that the outside air may become problematic.

Many people have reported in recent years that locations that used to feel terrific to them have suddenly become no-go areas.

Areas that might be treated with fire retardants seem to be particularly risky, but other factors can change things as well.

Many building techniques that seem promising in terms of prevention of toxic mold may be prohibited by local zoning.

For instance, non-traditional construction is not allowed in many locations.

In other locations, wall insulation of a certain type may be required.

Those mold avoiders who have considered what would be necessary to make a home wholly mold-safe have often reported that most architects and builders are very resistant to cooperating with them on this.

In addition, the use of special mold-resistant designs tends to make a house much more expensive than a regular house.

Although many mold avoiders state that they would be happy with a small home that would not be very expensive to build, zoning regulations very often have minimum size regulations.

A worst-case scenario to consider when building an expensive mold-safe house is that changes in air quality could make the home uninhabitable and that non-Moldies might be unwilling to pay anywhere near what the home cost to build.

Other risks are that toxic mold or other problematic substances will eventually render the home uninhabitable by the individual regardless of what efforts are made in the design and building stages.

Some individuals have reported that cross-contaminations with Hell Toxin have made previously good residences unlivable, for instance.

Other particularly problematic toxins that are even more difficult to manage have the possibility of emerging as well.

Another risk is that reactivities will change over time.

For instance, individuals who are starting out with avoidance have the potential of developing stronger reactivities to substances that currently seem only slightly problematic or of developing entirely new reactivities.

Eventually some individuals may become less reactive to certain substances or in general.

If any of these things occur, then a home that seems appropriate at one point in time may become less appropriate or less necessary later on.

Housing Decisions

In general, not making any long-term commitments with regard to housing tends to be a good idea for those just starting to pursue mold avoidance.

This is the case for signing long-term rental contracts and making purchases, and it is even more so for building specialty housing where the investment cannot be recouped if it doesn't work out.

Generally it takes people at least a few years after starting mold avoidance to have enough understanding of their reactions to be able to make any long-term commitments.

Even then, short-term commitments are safer.

Insofar as long-term commitments are required, choosing ones where the majority of the investment will not be lost if things do not go as hoped is a good idea.

This is the case with any kind of housing, whether it be a building, an RV, an automobile or even a tent.

In most cases, a rental situation is safest.

The purchase of an existing building that can be relatively easily resold is a possibility if there is a particular reason that it seems to be necessary.

In a few cases, building mold-safe housing from scratch may turn out to be the most appropriate solution.

This sometimes may be the case for people with very severe reactivities; for people with reactivities to a wide variety of molds (possibly including non-toxic molds); or for people with reactivities to a wide variety of other environmental substances.

Those individuals may require more control over their environments than any rental or purchase of an existing property may have the potential of giving them.

In that case, looking for a piece of property that is secluded from outside influences and that feels particularly good on which to build may be worth considering.

Even in that circumstance though, considering carefully the likelihood that the outdoor air possibly will become intolerable as well as the potential resale value may be worthwhile.

Building Styles

While there is no building style that is absolutely guaranteed to be safe for those who are hyperreactive to toxic mold, some styles are much more problematic than others.

Likely the worst possible style is the one used in the vast majority of homes built in the US and other modern countries over the past 40 years or so.

This style includes drywall, wall insulation, an HVAC system, pipes hidden in the wall, and relatively little indoor/outdoor air circulation.

Especially when combined with poor-quality construction, this is a recipe for the growth of Stachybotrys and other particularly toxic molds.

Following are some comments about alternative building styles that may be worth considering when buying or building.

* **Metal.** Metal buildings tend to be mold resistant, provided that drywall is not used inside. Some mold avoiders also like metal because it can be effectively treated with a flamethrower torch if it becomes cross-contaminated with particularly problematic toxins. Because it is lightweight, it may be appropriate for a tiny house built on a trailer bed. On the downside: metal buildings can be leaky, damp and – if not well insulated - particularly hot in summer and cold in winter.

* **Log or timber frame.** Although they are made of wood, these homes appear to be relatively resistant to the growth of toxic molds. The thick logs serve as good insulation, eliminating the need for additional wall insulation. Omitting the use of drywall and HVAC systems would make this kind of home even safer.

* **Adobe.** Traditional adobe homes have the same basic advantages of log homes. However, adobe homes tend to leak, meaning that the addition of drywall to an adobe can create a mold nightmare. Adobe homes using plaster or other non-cellulose materials for interior walls may be relatively safe.

* **Straw bale or cobb.** Stachybotrys sometimes grows on straw, and so the condition of the straw prior to the building of the home is important. Once the home is up, it may be relatively mold-resistant.

* **Concrete.** Rastra block construction or other concrete tends to be mold resistant, especially if drywall is not used.

* **Earthship.** These off-the-grid homes are constructed mainly of tires filled with dirt. Although they occasionally are reported as having non-toxic mold in them, toxic mold seems to be more uncommon.

* **Older homes.** Homes built prior to the 1970's sometimes may be very good in terms of mold growth. An important factor is whether they have been "improved" with the addition of drywall and wall insulation. Insofar as shredded newspapers have been used to fill the gaps between the inner and outer walls, they can be very bad indeed.

Following are some ways in which some mold avoiders have proposed altering modern building styles to make them more mold-safe.

* **Drywall alternatives.** Plaster (used in buildings prior to the 1970's) is resistant to mold growth and continues to be an alternative. A modern version is Plastermax. Magnesiacore is a drywall alternative that includes no cellulose. (Note: "Greenboard" meant to be used in bathrooms does contain cellulose and becomes moldy very easily.)

* **HVAC alternatives.** HVAC ductwork tends to be a breeding ground for toxic mold. Radiant heat, a wood stove or electric heat are alternatives.

* **Wall insulation.** The kind of design used in conventional homes (with condensation-producing plastic used to reduce air flow and mold-supporting insulation used between the exterior and interior walls) is best avoided.

* **Insulation alternatives.** Airkrete and styrofoam are insulations that do not become moldy when exposed to water.

* **Plumbing.** Having plumbing outside of walls rather than buried inside them would allow better monitoring for leaks.

* **Basements and crawl spaces.** Both of these tend to be problem spots with regard to toxic mold growth. Crawl spaces can be particularly problematic since water issues often can occur without anyone being aware. Avoiding these entirely or - at most - leaving the basement unfinished and empty may be a good idea.

* **Framework.** Most houses have wood framework. Considering that good wood has become more difficult for builders to obtain, metal framework may be a better idea if a frame home must be built.

* **Composite wood products.** Plywood and other similar products have substantial amounts of glues and other chemicals in them that may provide substrate for particularly problematic toxic mold growth. Avoiding these may be a good idea.

* **Ventilation.** Heat recovery ventilators are somewhat helpful in letting fresh air into a home, but air circulation in modern buildings still tends to be lower than desirable to reduce mold growth (especially between inside and outside walls).

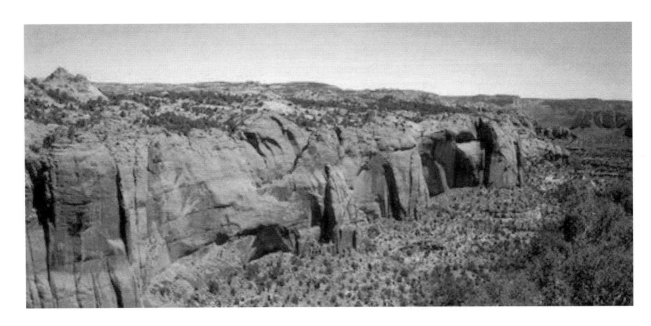

Navajo National Monument in northeastern Arizona.

Chapter 53

Testing & Remediation

Commercial testing of buildings has limitations and should be approached with care by those who believe or know that they are hyperreactive to toxic mold.

Those who are hyperreactive usually report that buildings that have been contaminated with super toxins or even substantial amounts of regular Stachybotrys are virtually impossible to remediate to the point that reactions do not occur.

Such homes usually can be remediated to the point that healthy individuals are able to live in them without getting sick, however.

It may be possible to remediate homes with less problematic ordinary toxic molds (such as Penicillium/Aspergillus) to the point where they are safe for mold avoiders, especially when the hyperreactivity is less severe.

Mold Testing

Many commonly used mold tests do not detect the presence of Stachybotrys in the environment.

These tests therefore can be misleading in terms of falsely reassuring people of the safety of a particular building and thus may be best avoided.

For instance, Stachybotrys does not generally grow on the inexpensive Petri dish tests sold at Home Depot and other mass retailers.

In addition, Stachybotrys produces a particularly heavy spore that falls quickly to the ground and then dissolves into spore fragments that mingle with other dust.

Rarely do the expensive air tests used by mold "professionals" pick up pictures of whole Stachy spores in the air, therefore.

The one test that may have some value in determining the extent to which a home contains problematic toxic mold is the Environmental Relative Moldiness Index (ERMI).

The ERMI was originally developed by the Environmental Protection Agency (EPA).

It looks at a dust sample from the environment to determine through genetic analysis the particular molds (toxic and non-toxic) present in the environment.

The cost in 2014 was about $300.

The ERMI index score provides information about how problematic the building is compared to other buildings in the US.

For instance, a score of 0 is stated to be an average home in terms of toxic mold, while a score of 15 is considered to be in the worst 10% of all buildings.

The ERMI is not a perfect test. It sometimes can miss the presence of substantial amounts of toxic mold growth entirely (especially if it is sealed inside a wall) and also does not distinguish especially problematic super toxins from regular toxins.

However, for those who are not yet clear enough to use their own reactions to determine the relative safety of various environments, the ERMI may provide some useful information as long as it is not assumed to be 100% accurate.

Getting clear enough to use one's own reactions to gauge environments always is a preferable to any standard test such as the ERMI.

The HERTSMI-2 test was developed by Dr. Ritchie Shoemaker based on looking at the ERMI results of the thousands of mold illness patients in his database.

It uses the same genetic testing as the ERMI but considers only five particularly problematic molds.

Shoemaker states that the test is particularly useful for allowing people who already have been made sick by toxic mold to determine if a new building is safe enough for them to occupy.

In 2014, the HERTSMI-2 was available for $125 from Mycometrics.

The HERTSMI-2 score also can be calculated from an ERMI result.

Mold-sniffing dogs have the potential of being extremely effective at finding hidden toxic mold in buildings, provided that they have been well-trained.

A downside is that dogs tend to be even more susceptible to the negative effects of toxic mold than humans, meaning that the dogs may be harmed by their work.

Relatively few mold dogs are available in the US, and they are even rarer in other countries.

Remediation

If a house is found through testing of whatever sort to be problematic in terms of toxic mold, the next question may be to figure out where the mold is hiding.

Insofar as a mold dog is not being used, probably the best way to make this determination is to hire someone very knowledgeable about toxic mold and building design to walk through the house and guess where all the problem spots might be.

A tool to measure the presence of humidity levels within the walls also may be helpful.

Then, under hazardous materials protocols, the suspect areas can be opened up and the mold safely removed.

This involves sealing off the area with a plastic barrier and then carefully removing and discarding all moldy materials in a safe way.

This needs to be done by professionals (or by other individuals fully versed in professional techniques).

Individuals who are hyperreactive to toxic mold should not be present when the work is being done.

Mold Hot Spots

Although mold can grow in a wide variety of places in buildings, following are some of the most typical problem areas.

* Roof failures.

* Wall insulation (especially cellulose such as newspaper) combined with leaks.

* Pipe leaks in drywall.

* Showers. (Often tile backing or "green board" will become moldy even from condensation.)

* Flooring failures. (This may often be caused by carpets being washed or otherwise getting wet and then drying slowly.)

* House improperly built. (Some homes are moldy before they even go on the market.)

* Window leaks.

* Duct systems not maintained.

* Condensation interface (generally the north wall).

* Flooding.

* Crawl spaces and basements.

Ozone

Ozone has the ability to kill mold in an environment.

It also has been shown to have the ability to degrade mold toxins, though this takes much more time than killing mold.

Quality remediators agree that ozone is not the solution to any environmental mold problem.

Killing mold (rather than removing it intact) tends to make toxic mold problems worse, since dead colonies tend to release more of their spores into the air than live ones do.

Although the use of ozone may eventually degrade mold toxins to some extent, this usually is incomplete.

The use of strong ozone also may volatilize chemicals, degrade plastic and harm electronics items in a home.

Some mold avoiders have reported that subsequent to the proper remediation of their homes via mold removal, the extended use of strong ozone has allowed the space to feel somewhat better to them.

Ozone also may have the ability to destroy whole spores, making it less likely that new colonies will emerge if a new water event occurs.

We have virtually no reports of successful mold avoiders reporting that ozone has made particularly problematic spaces tolerable for them, however.

Ozone can be very damaging to lungs or even deadly if it is breathed, and so people and animals need to be away from the environment when it is running.

Hydroxyl generators work somewhat similarly to ozone generators, but the reactions take place in the machine rather than in the environment.

They work more slowly than ozone and are primarily used for odor control.

The extent to which they may be helpful with regard to mold toxins is unknown.

Part 7

SOCIAL ASPECTS

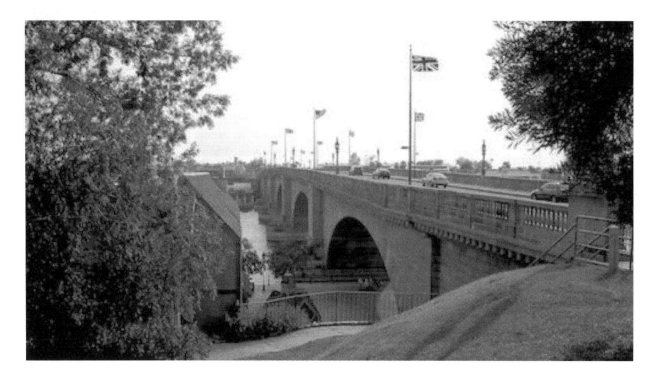

The old London Bridge (transported from England) in Lake Havasu, Arizona.

Chapter 54

Rebuilding a Life

Rebuilding a rewarding life within the constraints of mold avoidance can be a challenge.

Still, many mold avoiders have reported success in doing that.

Following are some basic approaches that mold avoiders have found to work for them, either for short periods of time or on a more permanent basis.

Staying with Friends

Insofar as family or friends have a home that is reasonably tolerable, staying with them for a while has the potential of providing shelter while individuals seek out a more permanent situation.

Very often staying with family or friends does not work, however.

For instance, many mold avoiders have found their parents' home to be particularly problematic (which makes some sense since exposures during childhood may have contributed to their becoming sick later in life).

Staying with family and friends in the same geographic location will not provide a break from outdoor problems that may be a factor for those who are particularly ill.

In several cases, those affected by Hell Toxin have reported needing to actively avoid the homes of people who they have visited in the past because of cross-contamination.

Still, for those who can tolerate the homes of friends or relatives, they could provide a safe harbor for at least a while.

Residence Rentals

Many individuals pursuing mold avoidance have had successful experiences renting houses or apartments.

The main upside to this approach is that it seems a lot like a normal life.

Particularly for individuals with families, it can be a good choice.

The downside is the lack of control that people often have over rentals.

It is hard to make sure that the property is being maintained in ways that do not result in mold growth or chemical exposures.

Especially in apartments, activities of neighbors (such as their bringing in cross-contaminated possessions or using chemicals) may be a problem as well.

As a result, those who choose to live in rentals tend to spend a great deal of time wondering if they are reacting to something in their environment, trying to figure out what that thing might be, and negotiating with landlords or neighbors to address or prevent problems.

Because environments have the potential of becoming intolerable, not committing to a long-term lease is important for those pursuing mold avoidance.

Options to obtain a short-term lease may include paying more on a monthly basis or having a clause that states that the lease can be broken with a doctor's note.

Choosing a home with a balcony, a porch or a yard where a tent can be put up is a strategy used successfully by a number of mold avoiders to get more access to fresh air.

Buying a House

A few mold avoiders have done well in houses that they have purchased.

Others have had very unhappy experiences where problems that could not be remediated well enough for their tolerance level have emerged.

With few exceptions, it is very difficult to ensure that any conventional home will not develop problems that will be impossible to remediate to the standard required by those who are hyperreactive.

Therefore, whether the home likely will be able to be resold easily to a healthy person without a loss is a key consideration when considering purchasing.

A House with an MECU

Some people (especially those who are very reactive) may find it difficult or impossible to find any house or apartment that feels good enough for them to live in on a full-time basis.

While they may be able to spend limited amounts of time in certain homes, sleeping in them on a regular basis may drive them further down the power curve.

Certain MECU options (such as a converted cargo trailer or a thoroughly off-gassed Camplite) may be much more tolerable for these individuals.

In that case, parking a good MECU outside of a somewhat tolerable home may allow a compromise that allows some of the conveniences of having a home but provides a more pristine sleeping environment.

Although it likely will be more expensive to rent a house than to rent a spot in an RV park, it also is possible that having access to bathroom and kitchen facilities in the home will allow a more basic RV to suffice.

The backyard of a house also can be helpful for mold avoidance activities, such as periodically sleeping in a tent to get more clear or hanging laundry to dry.

This approach may be particularly appropriate for those with families.

In that case, the house may provide a location for everyone to spend time together, while the MECU may allow the reactive individual(s) to get clearer on a regular basis.

In cases where people have obliging relatives or friends who live in a semi-tolerable home in a place with good outdoor air, parking an RV outside the home and then using their bathroom and kitchen could be a reasonable long-term solution.

An alternative to an MECU in areas with relatively warm weather year round is to sleep in a sheltered outdoor area such as a gazebo.

A temporary solution is for reactive individuals to plan to sleep in a tent outside a semi-tolerable house.

Although many people have slept in a backyard tent for limited periods of time, weather and frustration issues tend to make it less suitable for the long-term.

The Homestead

This approach involves purchasing a piece of property (often in a remote area) and building a mold-safe house and other amenities on it.

This may be especially appropriate for individuals who are very reactive to a variety of substances and have a hard time living in regular civilization.

It also may be more appropriate than living in an MECU for those who need space to work or who have families.

Some individuals creating this kind of setup consider the possibility of offering accommodations to other mold avoiders, with the goal of using rent to offset some of the expenses.

The main advantage to this kind of approach is that it provides a greater degree of control than other non-mobile living options.

A disadvantage is that this type of setup may be quite expensive to make operational and may be difficult to sell if the need or desire occurs to move on.

Living in a Vehicle

Not infrequently, individuals are driven from their homes by toxic mold and cannot find an alternative home that they can afford or tolerate.

Some of those individuals end up living in their vehicles for at least a while, until they can figure out other options.

A van may be more suitable for this type of living than other vehicles.

In some cases, especially in scenic areas in the western half of the US, living out of a vehicle is considered somewhat acceptable.

It still may be better to take the stance when asked of being on an extended road trip rather than homeless, however.

In many other places, living out of a vehicle other than an RV is frowned upon both socially and legally.

Therefore, especially if individuals plan to park on the street or in public parking lots, they may need to concern themselves with issues of stealth.

Having local access to a shower and a place to prepare food may be very helpful for people pursuing this approach in civilization rather than camping areas.

RV Park Living

Especially in the western half of the US, many people live full-time in their RV's in RV parks.

Some of these are snowbirds, alternating between locations as the seasons change. Others live in a single place year round.

Although many RV parks are basic, some cater to affluent individuals and can be very deluxe.

The cost tends to range from $300-700 per month.

Some parks have no bathroom facilities, have moldy bathrooms, or require that guests have holding tanks in their RV's.

Therefore, individuals who do not have plumbing in their RV's may be more limited in terms of the choices available to them.

One issue with living in RV parks is that many RV's have substantial toxic mold problems and can be bothersome to mold avoiders parked nearby.

Having the ability to park near other long-term vehicles that feel okay or to move within the park if necessary may be helpful to keep this issue from becoming a major problem.

On the Road

Many mold avoiders have spent extensive amounts of time traveling around the US or other locations while camping in their tents, vehicles or RV's.

Spending extended periods of time at sea on a boat would fit into this category as well.

An advantage of traveling around for mold avoiders is that they get to see how they feel in different locations.

As a result, they may become more skilled at avoidance and also eventually may hit upon an optimal place to settle down permanently.

In addition, traveling around sometimes can provide a boost to the spirits of individuals who have become discouraged from mold illness.

On the downside, depending on how it is done, traveling can end up being more expensive than staying in one place.

Traveling also tends to be more suitable for people who are not as sick or who already have regained some of their health.

Meeting specific dietary needs or other special needs can be more challenging when traveling than when staying in one place.

Some people may start to feel psychologically adrift when they have traveled around for an extensive period of time.

Many people who are pursuing this approach frequently stay in hotels or cabins as a change of pace.

Settling down for a few weeks or a month in a particularly good campground or an RV park may provide more of a feeling of being grounded as well.

A Note on Entertaining

While many people enjoy entertaining at home, this introduces the possibility that guests will inadvertently introduce particularly problematic toxins into the home.

Unless friends and family are willing to go through decontamination procedures before entering the designated safe space, it may be better to spend time with them somewhere other than the home environment.

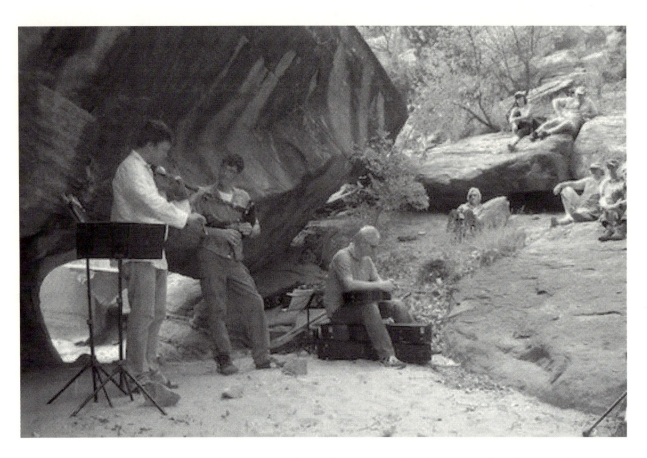

A Moab Musical Festival concert performed at Canyonlands National Park in Utah.

Chapter 55

Managing the Responses of Others

While toxic mold illness is becoming increasingly accepted as a legitimate phenomenon, there still are many people who have never heard of it or who are skeptical about whether it is an actual physiological problem.

Although toxic mold hyperreactivity has been experienced by many individuals, it has yet to be studied in a systematic way and is less well-known than reactivities to various human-made chemicals.

The idea of improving health by systematically avoiding even tiny amounts of toxic mold is even less well-known.

Therefore, individuals pursuing mold avoidance generally can anticipate encountering some challenges with regard to successfully navigating interpersonal relationships.

Following are some thoughts related to handling these.

Family

Having the support of partners and other close family members can be extremely helpful for those who want to pursue mold avoidance successfully.

However, even the most loving and supportive family members can be very resistant to the idea that mold avoidance may be worth pursuing.

In most cases, this is at least in part because they fear the consequences with regard to their relationship, their family and their current life.

When family members have had the same exposure as the individual who is sick, they also may be concerned at a deep (even unconscious) level about what this may mean for their own health.

Leaving a bad environment and pursuing mold avoidance can be life-altering from a variety of perspectives - practical, emotional and financial.

It therefore should not be a surprise that family members might be resistant to the idea.

In addition, affected individuals who are considering starting mold avoidance usually are being affected emotionally by toxic exposures and also are justifiably anxious about what might be ahead for them.

This may put stress on relationships.

In many cases, mold avoiders have reported that developing a clear plan on their own of what they want to happen and then working to obtain buy-in from family members has had positive results.

Sharing information about other people's experiences and about the opinions of doctors also may be helping in persuading family members that mold illness is a real phenomenon and that avoidance may be helpful.

Although it can be difficult for new mold avoiders to remain loving and reasonable and patient in their interactions with their family members, doing so may be helpful as well.

Friends & Acquaintances

Whether to talk about mold reactivity or mold avoidance with friends and acquaintances is a personal decision.

In most cases, even if people are skeptical of whether the reactivity is real, no real harm will result.

However, those individuals who are not currently attached to a house or apartment may want to be careful with regard to sharing that information with others that they do not know well and trust.

Biases against homelessness can be very strong, and even campgrounds may make a special effort to keep out those individuals that they believe to be homeless.

Employers

Many mold avoiders find it challenging to find employment in an environment that is good enough for them.

Even if employers really want particular individuals to be working for them, they may be at a loss with regard to how to make buildings good enough for them.

In general, a good strategy may be to figure out a solution that would seem to be workable for both parties and then to make a case to the employer about why it is a good idea.

For instance, this may involve a move to a different building or a different part of the building.

In some cases, asking for accommodations to work from home - possibly even from a different part of the country - may be an acceptable solution.

Freelancing from home (possibly through an online site such as ODesk.com or Elance.com) may be another way for some individuals to work if they cannot find an office building that is good enough for them.

Landlords

Mold avoiders' reports suggest that a high percentage of landlords tend to be wary of individuals who have issues with toxic mold or various chemicals.

Toxic mold in buildings is something that can be very difficult to control even if a landlord is doing everything right.

Many landlords believe that it would be difficult to run their properties without using various chemicals that might be objectionable to those with sensitivities.

Some landlords have had negative experiences with individuals who are sensitive to mold or chemicals raising objections to how they run their properties.

Keeping this in mind when interacting with landlords thus may be worthwhile.

This especially may be the case prior to signing a lease.

In many cases, a landlord who decides that a particular potential tenant is likely to be too much trouble may decide to rent to someone else instead - an unfortunate occurrence since tolerable homes may be very hard to come by.

Some mold avoiders have concluded that it is better to say nothing about their mold reactivity to their landlords.

Although mold avoiders usually want to obtain a short-term lease, there usually are many other legitimate reasons for asking for this other than fears that the place may become problematic with regard to mold or chemicals.

If an ERMI test is to be done, it may be necessary to inform the landlord.

However, many landlords may react better if it is stated that this is just a precaution "because someone I know got sick from mold" rather than a primary requirement.

Landlords have more control over chemical usage than they do about mold growth.

Asking in a casual way before signing the lease what kinds of chemicals are used in the facility may be a good idea.

If those chemicals are wholly unacceptable, then discussing the situation more frankly to see if accommodations can be made could be worth a try.

A very few legal cases suggest that chemical sensitivities may be covered under the Americans with Disabilities Act (ADA), and conceivably this could be used as leverage (in conjunction with a doctor's note) to encourage landlords not to use certain chemicals.

In practice, many landlords seem to believe that it is unlikely that they will be harmed by a lawsuit related to this matter and therefore are not accommodating when individuals use this tactic.

Schools

A high percentage of US schools are problematic enough with regard to toxic mold to cause problems even for healthy individuals.

Even if children have survived a mold exposure and appear to be mostly well, avoidance of particularly problematic school buildings may be a good idea in terms of protecting them from future illness.

In many cases, school administrators know that toxic mold is a health hazard but do not have the money to fix the problem.

Asking for accommodations with regard to the child being allowed to attend a different school in the same district may have some potential of being accepted.

Some mold avoiders choose to homeschool their children, in large part to keep them out of moldy school buildings.

Physicians

Most physicians know nothing about toxic mold illness and have many misconceptions about chronic multisystem illnesses.

They tend to be disbelieving about the idea that individuals can be very ill as a result of exposures to toxic mold.

The idea that people can be hyperreactive to toxic mold and benefit from avoidance of it likely will at best be viewed by them under the framework of its being an allergy.

Although in many cases having chronic multisystem disease is very relevant to the types of treatments that patients should and should not receive, the majority of doctors do not understand enough about the illness to give proper treatments.

Therefore, having a trusted doctor who is familiar with chronic multisystem illness for phone consults or in-person visits can be helpful.

Despite the fact that most non-specialist doctors are unfamiliar with the role that toxic mold can play in illness, they still may in some cases respond better to the idea of toxic mold poisoning than they do the illness being defined as ME/CFS, chronic Lyme disease or fibromyalgia.

Part 8

Appendices

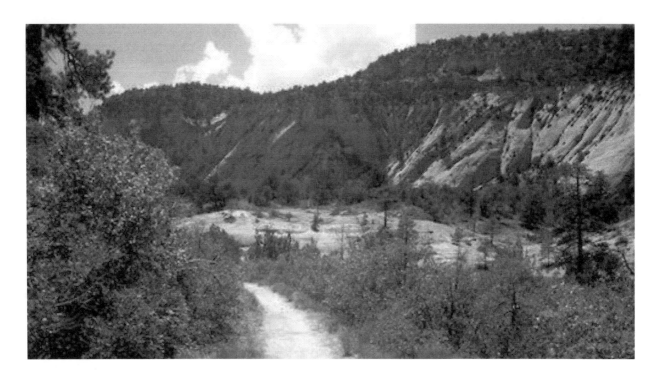

A hiking trail in southwestern Utah.

Appendix 1

Chronic Multisystem Disease

Following are is a discussion of the apparent role of mold toxicity and mold avoidance in some chronic multisystem illnesses.

Myalgic Encephalomyelitis

This is a disease in which individuals often first succumb suddenly to a "weird flu-like illness." Classic flu symptoms generally are present, but additional symptoms may include severe cognitive impairment, dizziness, temporarily paralysis, lack of coordination, and strong emotional feelings that have little to do with what is actually going on. In some cases, a herpes virus infection (such as EBV, herpes zoster or HHV6) may be diagnosed.

In many cases, this acute illness turns into myalgic encephalomyelitis, a disease with a specific set of symptoms and expected laboratory abnormalities.

This diagnosis is currently recognized by the US government as part of what it calls "chronic fatigue syndrome (ME/CFS)."

Anecdotally, the acute illness often (possibly always) occurs when a mold-susceptible individual has an encounter with a substantial amount of what has been dubbed the Mystery Toxin (see Chapter 30).

Very often, individuals who succumb acutely after exposure to this substance have been exposed on a regular basis to homes or workplaces that are particularly problematic with indoor toxic mold.

Usually they were already demonstrating some symptoms related to the disease long before acquiring the "flu-like illness."

One possibility is that the exposure to these toxins cause long-term damage to the immune system, allowing herpes-family viruses and other infections to run amuck.

Another possibility is that the fungus or other microorganism making the Mystery Toxin has the ability to colonize the human system and create ongoing effects.

Creating even more confusion, many individuals end up looking indistinguishable from the acute-onset patients even though their onset is much more gradual.

Anecdotally, those patients tend to also be living in homes that are particularly problematic with indoor toxic mold but have less upfront exposure to the Mystery Toxin than the acute onset patients generally do.

Many individuals qualifying for an ME diagnosis have found that they are hyperreactive to mold toxins and have benefited from the techniques discussed in this book.

Chronic Fatigue Syndrome

Chronic fatigue syndrome has been recognized by the CDC since 1988.

It originally was associated with an acute outbreak of ME in the Lake Tahoe area as well as what was then called chronic EBV syndrome.

Very recently, the government has taken to referring to the syndrome as "chronic fatigue syndrome (ME/CFS)."

However, as chronic fatigue syndrome is currently defined by the CDC, most individuals who consider themselves to have chronic multisystem illnesses with a different names (such as chronic Lyme disease, toxic mold illness, Gulf War illness or fibromyalgia) would qualify for a CFS diagnosis.

Many of those individuals would qualify for an ME diagnosis as well.

Many individuals qualifying for a CFS diagnosis report being hyperreactive to toxic mold, and most (but not all) of those who have tried mold avoidance according to the precepts in this book say that they have benefited from it.

Chronic Lyme Disease

Acute Lyme disease is a bacterial infection, caused by the tick-borne pathogen borrelia burgdorferi.

Usually it is resolved through treatment with antibiotics.

However, a minority of individuals who fall ill with Lyme disease after a tick bite do not fully recover even with antibiotic treatment.

This especially may be likely to occur if treatment is delayed.

This condition is officially called post Lyme disease syndrome by the CDC, but it frequently is referred to as chronic Lyme disease.

Patients with chronic Lyme tend to be very similar (in terms of laboratory test results, symptoms and illness course) to those who qualify for diagnoses of ME/CFS, Gulf War illness or toxic mold illness.

Why the illness does not resolve with antibiotics in these patients and what the relationship is between this illness and other chronic multisystem illnesses are important questions that have yet to be answered.

One hypothesis is that the toxins produced by borrelia may act similarly to mold toxins in causing neurological damage, immune dysfunction and systemic inflammation.

Insofar as certain individuals are unable to effectively eliminate these toxins from their systems, they might experience long-term health issues as a result.

Certain other microorganisms that often are "co-infections" with borrelia also produce toxins that could contribute to toxic overload if they are not effectively eliminated from the system.

Anecdotally, many individuals who acquired chronic Lyme disease subsequent to a tick bite report being hyperreactive to mold toxins.

These individuals very often have HLA DR genotypes that may make them more susceptible to toxic mold.

Frequently they report that they were living or working in buildings that were particularly problematic with regard to toxic mold when they first came down with the Lyme infection.

Possibly the immune compromising effects of the mold exposure makes people less likely to be able to get the Lyme disease under control.

Many individuals with chronic Lyme have tried mold avoidance and benefited from it.

Toxic Mold Illness

Significant scientific study has been done looking at the ability of water-damaged buildings with microbial growth to cause illness related to neurological and immune system damage.

Dr. Ritchie Shoemaker has a panel of laboratory tests that he states are indicative of individuals who have been made ill from these environments.

He calls the condition chronic inflammatory response syndrome (CIRS).

Individuals with ME and similar serious illnesses usually come up as meeting Shoemaker's criteria for a CIRS diagnosis.

The idea that moldy buildings can cause multisystem illness has become increasingly recognized in courts and within the scientific community.

However, neither toxic mold illness nor CIRS are as of yet recognized by US governmental agencies such as the CDC or NIH.

Nor are they recognized by governmental agencies of other countries.

Generally, individuals defining themselves as having these conditions became aware of mold in their home or work environments and consider it a primary cause of their illness.

The extent to which people with similar conditions using different names to describe their illness also unknowingly became sick in moldy homes or workplaces has never been formally studied.

Anecdotally, a high percentage of those individuals who have concluded that they were made ill by mold report that they are hyperreactive to it, and many of these have benefited from mold avoidance.

Gulf War Illness

Gulf War illness is similar to all the previously discussed illnesses with regard to symptoms, laboratory tests and illness course.

A main difference is to be where these individuals got sick (during military service) and that toxins of various sorts tend to be accepted as a possible cause of GWI.

Several GWI sufferers have reported being hyperreactive to toxic mold and have benefited from mold avoidance.

Fibromyalgia

Fibromyalgia is a disease that overlaps to a large degree with ME and the other previously discussed illnesses.

In addition, the vast majority of fibromyalgia sufferers would qualify for a CFS diagnosis, as described by the CDC.

Fibromyalgia and ME sufferers tend to have basically the same symptoms but in somewhat differing degrees.

With fibromyalgia, the emphasis is foremost on pain, with other symptoms secondary.

With ME, the emphasis tends to be much more on post-exertional malaise, which puts strict limits on the amount of activity that individuals can do without getting worse.

Some fibromyalgia sufferers do not experience as much post-exertional malaise and may benefit from exercise (especially exercise involving stretching).

However, many individuals who state that they have fibromyalgia would amply qualify for a diagnosis of ME.

Many fibromyalgia patients have reported being hyperreactive to toxic mold.

In combination with other treatments, quite a few fibromyalgia patients have reported benefiting from mold avoidance.

Multiple Chemical Sensitivity

People with multiple chemical sensitivity are by definition reactive to a variety of environmental chemicals.

The condition is often called environmental illness (EI).

Neither MCS nor EI is as of yet recognized by the US government or its agencies (such as the CDC).

A high percentage of people with MCS would qualify for a CFS definition, as the CDC has defined it.

Many would qualify for an ME diagnosis as well.

Some individuals with MCS or EI report that they first became ill in a problematic environment with regard to toxic mold.

It is unknown what percentage of MCS or EI sufferers were being exposed to problematic amounts or types of toxic mold when their illnesses began, however.

Many individuals with severe MCS have made active efforts to seek out better environments with regard to the chemical toxins that they know are bothering them, but in some cases remain quite ill.

Anecdotally, many of these individuals have been observed to be carrying around super toxins on their belongings, providing a possible explanation for why they make relatively little progress.

Many individuals identifying with the diagnoses of EI or MCS state that they are hyperreactive to mold toxins and that they benefit from avoiding these toxins.

Autism

Autism is a disease with many of the same issues as the other diseases described above.

Some researchers (such as the late Rich van Konynenburg) have posited that the main difference between ME/CFS and autism is that in autism, the brain damage occurs earlier in development and thus manifests differently.

The neonatal administration of certain aquatic biotoxins (such as domoic acid) in laboratory mammals creates a condition that looks a great deal like autism.

Symptoms resulting from administration of this toxin emerge well after birth and include learning and memory deficits, reduced seizure thresholds, aversion to novelty, social withdrawal, lowered activity level, increased perseveration, motor seizures characterized by scratching or swimming motions, lowered interest in nicotine, superior choice ability in completing mazes, changes in the dentate gyrus and hippocampus of the brain, and a mechanism that seems to be related to voltage-dependent calcium channels.

Neonatals are particularly susceptible to this toxin because of their incomplete blood-brain barrier. Often they are severely affected without the mother showing any signs of being harmed by the toxin.

Since what has been called the "Mystery Toxin" manifests in adults with ME similarly to domoic acid, a possible hypothesis in terms of causality is that autistic individuals have been exposed to this toxin while still in the womb.

A number of parents of children with autism have suggested that their children are especially hyperreactive to toxic mold, and many individuals who would qualify for an Asperger's diagnosis have benefited from avoidance.

Insofar as individuals with autism have a difficult time verbalizing their reactions, this may make it more difficult to help them to get clear enough to practice mold avoidance effectively.

Anecdotally, many parents of autistic children have chronic multisystem illness themselves and therefore may be reactive enough that they could learn to identify problematic toxins.

Objective measures such as the monitoring of heart rate or blood pressure also may be helpful in identifying problematic environments.

Amyotrophic Lateral Sclerosis

ALS (also called Lou Gehrig's disease or motor neurone disease) is increasingly accepted by scientists as a biotoxin-related illness.

One factor in the illness has been reported to be exposure to certain cyanobacteria manufacturing a potent toxin called BMAA.

ALS is a deadly disease with relatively few sufferers, but a few individuals with the disease have reported being especially hyperreactive to toxic mold.

Whether scrupulous avoidance of problematic environmental biotoxins would be helpful to them is as of yet unknown.

Multiple Sclerosis

Multiple sclerosis (MS) has been reported in the medical literature as having a particular association with gliotoxin, a mold toxin.

MS also seems to have a connection to Lyme disease.

For instance, the HLA DR genotype reported to be associated with chronic Lyme is in the literature as a risk factor for getting MS.

Some MS patients test positive on Lyme tests and report that their MS symptoms improve subsequent to Lyme treatment.

An unpublished but interesting study looking at Lyme deaths and MS deaths suggests that the same locations have particularly high death rates for both diseases.

(A high percentage of these locations also are ones where the Mystery Toxin has been reported to be particularly problematic by mold avoiders.)

MS is acknowledged to be less of an issue in places that mold avoiders often report to be good locations, such as islands near the equator.

It thus seems possible that MS patients might benefit from mold avoidance, though we have yet to receive reports on this being tried.

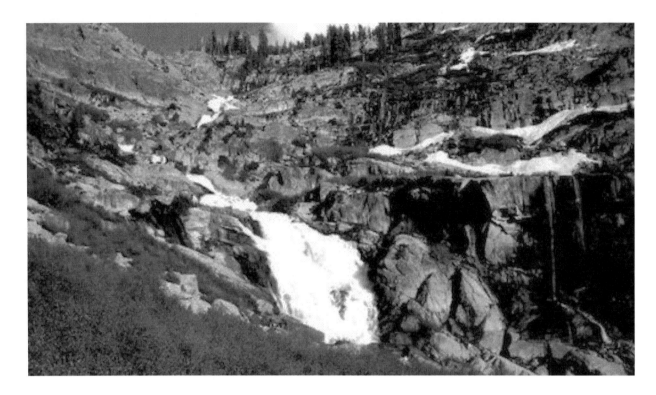

A waterfall at Sequoia National Park in California.

Appendix 2

Glossary

Above Tolerance. An environment (particularly a home or work environment) that is host to a larger amount of mycotoxins than a particular individual can bear without becoming ill.

Adsorbed. The process by which mycotoxins (or other gases or liquids) bond permanently to the surface of a solid item.

Aflatoxin. A mycotoxin present in food and buildings that has been shown in the literature to be a cause of liver cancer.

Agitated Exhaustion. A state experienced by CFS sufferers as a result of their being unable to sleep deeply or restfully; may be caused by the presence of mold toxins.

Air Test. Environmental test looking for the presence of mold spores in the air; not helpful in gauging the presence of Stachybotrys.

Ambiently Bad. A place that causes a mold reactor to suffer a decline in mood.

Aspergillus. A toxic mold that is easily airborne, contaminates food and sometimes colonizes the human body.

Avoidance. Staying away from areas or objects contaminated with toxic mold spores, spore fragments or mycotoxins.

Bad Building. A building with a problematic level of mold toxicity.

Bad Zone. An area problematic for mold responders.

Balance the Books. Spend time in a low-mold area in order to mitigate the effects of previous mold exposures.

Benign Mold. Fungi that do not manufacture mycotoxins.

Berkeley Toxin. Another name for Mystery Toxin.

Biotoxin. Toxin made by certain organisms, including certain types of mold, certain strains of Lyme bacteria, brown recluse spiders, certain types of algae, certain dinoflagellates and certain other bacteria.

Biowarfare Protocols. Methods used to combat the effects of biological, chemical and radiological weapons, using the principles of "detect, evacuate, avoid and decontaminate."

Black Mold. Another name for Stachybotrys chartarum.

Blood-Brain Barrier (BBB). A boundary surrounding the brain that prevents the penetration of certain substances such as commonly used chemicals; satratoxin can increase its permeability.

Blue-Sky Day. A clear sunny day with a low level of outdoor toxic mold.

Brain Fog. Decreased cognitive abilities experienced by Chronic Fatigue Syndrome and mycotoxin illness sufferers.

Breaking the Response. Spending an extended amount of time in an environment with a low level of toxic mold, in order to bring down a complement spike.

Camplite. A trailer containing no wood that has been used successfully by a number of mold avoiders.

Carrying the Response. Having hair or clothing contaminated by previous exposures to toxic mold spores or spore fragments.

Casita. A fiberglass trailer brand made in Rice, Texas.

Cholestyramine (CSM). A medication that was originally used to lower cholesterol and that is effective at removing mycotoxins and other biotoxins from the body.

Chronic multisystem disease (or illness). A category of illness consisting of myalgic encephalomyelitis, chronic fatigue syndrome, chronic Lyme disease, fibromyalgia, Gulf War illness and other related conditions.

Clear. A system that is free enough of toxic mold for complement to decrease to normal levels, or an area that is low enough in toxic mold for this to occur in a particular individual.

Colony. A growth of mold.

Compensation. Spending time in areas low in toxic mold in order to be able to tolerate greater toxic mold exposure at other times.

Converted Cargo Trailer. A utility trailer with added amenities to make it more livable as an RV.

Contamination. The exposure of an item to toxic mold spores or spore fragments, causing it to carry mycotoxins on it.

Cross Contaminated (or Contaminated). The extent to which an object or individual is carrying potentially detrimental toxins.

Cross Contamination. The process by which toxic mold spores or spore fragments dislodge themselves from one item and attach themselves to another item.

Cyanobacteria. A microorganism that generally grows on water and that has the potential of producing toxins.

Damp Down. The decrease in complement to a normal level as a result of decreases in toxic mold exposures.

Decontaminate (Decon). Wash one's hair, take a shower and change clothes after being exposed to toxic mold spores or spore fragments.

Delayed Response. Negative reactions experienced hours or days after mycotoxin exposures occur.

Denature. The process by which items contaminated with mycotoxins become more tolerable to mold responders.

Dent Test. Observing the extent to which skin indentations as a result of pressure occur and persist as a way in which to measure the extent to which mycotoxins have created hypoperfusion or edema, and thus affected the system as a whole.

Depression Response (also Anger/Anxiety/Panic/Suicide Response). A negative change in mood resulting from exposure to mycotoxins.

"Desert." A wilderness area with a low level of toxic mold.

Detoxification. The process by which toxic chemicals of any sort are expelled from the body.

Die Down. The process by which items contaminated by toxic mold lose their ability to negatively affect mold responders.

Dormant Spores. Mold spores that have the potential of growing into new colonies if water and a food source is obtained.

Down-regulate. A decrease in inflammation to a normal level, accomplished as a result of decreased exposure to toxic mold or other problematic substances.

Dose Related. An effect determined by the total amount of toxic mold to which a person has been exposed.

Duration Related. An effect determined by the length of time that a person has been exposed to toxic mold.

Effect. The changes that occur in the systems of sufferers of CFS or mold illness as a result of environmental exposures to toxic mold and/or related substances.

EMF's. Electromagnetic fields such as those emitted by satellites, cellular phones, power lines, CD players and computers; have the potential to cause molds to release more toxins or more potent toxins.

EMF Sensitivity. Being negatively affected by electromagnetic fields such as those emitted by satellites, cellular phones, power lines, CD players and computers.

Environmental Mold. Mold found in indoor or outdoor air.

ERMI. Environmental test looking at the presence of genetic material from molds.

Erythropoietin (Epo). An anti-cytokine protein that can improve VEGF problems in CFS and mycotoxin illness sufferers; may be increased by temporarily spending time at high altitudes or through administration of the drug Procrit.

Exposure. Coming into contact with toxic mold spores, spore fragments or poisons.

Extreme Responder (or Extreme Reactor). An individual who experiences negative symptoms as a result of exposure to very small amounts of mycotoxins.

Fusarium. A common outdoor mold that often produces trichothecenes.

Get Clear. Going to a low-mold area in order to reduce the symptoms of previous mycotoxin exposures.

Gluten Intolerance. Negative reactions to consuming protein found in wheat, barley, rye and oats; may dissipate when mycotoxin reactivity is successfully addressed through avoidance.

Godforsaken Desert (or Godforsaken Wilderness). Any area far from civilization and with a very low level of toxic mold.

Good Day/Bad Day Phenomenon. A common tendency of CFS sufferers to feel better on some days than others, related in at least some cases to the total amount of toxic mold in the air.

Hell Toxin (or Hell Fire Toxin). As reported by many mold avoiders, a particularly damaging toxin that is especially potent at causing burning or other skin issues.

HEPA Filter. An air filter that removes mold spores from the air, but that does not provide protection from small spore fragments or the mycotoxins manufactured by toxic mold.

High Spore Count Day. A day with a high level of outdoor toxic mold.

Hit. Contact with mold toxins.

Hit the Wall. Reaching a level of toxic mold exposure that causes the individual to suffer debilitating effects lasting for an extended length of time, and that cannot be quickly reversed by subsequent exposure to pristine areas.

HLA DR. A genetic test that can be used to assess an individual's ability to effectively eliminate from the body mycotoxins, Lyme toxins and other biotoxins, as well as tendency toward low MSH production.

HERTSMI-2. An environmental mold test similar to the ERMI and developed by Dr. Ritchie Shoemaker.

Herxheimer. An exacerbation of symptoms due to increased cytokine effects in Lyme patients taking antibiotics or cholestyramine.

Hyperreactive. Being affected by very small amounts of toxic mold to a much more dramatic extent than the average person, due to complement activation.

Hypoperfusion. Decreased blood flow through an organ (including the skin), a problem common amongst CFS and mycotoxin poisoning sufferers and caused by low levels of VEGF.

Ick (Idiopathic Contaminant or IC). Another name for Mystery Toxin.

Intensification Reaction (or Intensification Response). Phenomenon in which an individual's reactivity to toxic mold increases dramatically after spending time in a place with a relatively low level of toxic mold.

Ionophore Toxins. A lipid-soluble molecule (including those made by toxic mold) that transports materials across cell membranes and thus distributes them evenly throughout the body.

Itch Toxin. Another name for Hell Toxin.

Locations Effect. The tendency of CFS sufferers to feel better in some places than others; may be related to outdoor toxic mold levels.

Low Spore Count Day. A day with a low level of outdoor toxic mold.

Lyme Disease. An acute or chronic illness caused by several species of bacteria belonging to the genus Borrelia and characterized by a wide variety of physical, cognitive and emotional symptoms (some similar to those attributable to mycotoxins).

Lyme Susceptible Genotype. HLA DR category that indicates an individual who is unable to easily detoxify Lyme toxins from the system.

Lymie. Individual suffering from Lyme disease, especially chronic Lyme disease.

Masking. Compensations made by the system in order to continue to function despite toxic exposures; can prevent the recognition that an overload is occurring.

MCS. Multiple Chemical Sensitivity, a condition in which sufferers respond negatively to a wide variety of chemicals that do not affect most people; may abate with successful avoidance of toxic mold.

Mildew. Superficial growth of fungi on surfaces.

Mobile Environmental Containment Unit (MECU). Recreational vehicle or other vehicle that can be used for showering after mold contamination and for flexibility in being able to travel to areas that are low in toxic mold at a particular time.

Mold. Any of various fungi that often cause disintegration of organic matter; may be used as shorthand for "toxic mold" or "mycotoxins."

Mold Allergy. The body's reaction to the misidentification of benign mold as problematic; characterized by symptoms such as sneezing, watery eyes, stuffy nose, itching or asthma.

Mold Avoider. An individual who makes an effort to obtain wellness by avoiding toxic mold.

Moldie. An individual who suffers from negative effects of toxic mold, especially from very small amounts of toxic mold.

Mold Responder. An individual who suffers from negative effects of toxic mold.

Mold Avoidance Sabbatical. A finite period of time spent in a wilderness area very low in toxic mold, in order to gauge mold reactivity, increase mold sensitivity and/or promote healing.

Mold Susceptible Genotype. HLA DR category that indicates an individual who is unable to easily detoxify mycotoxins from the system.

Mold Toxicity. Poisoning resulting from toxic mold exposures

Mold Unfriendly Environment. A building or vehicle designed to prevent the growth of toxic mold.

Mold Zone. An area that constantly or frequently is hit with a large amount of airborne toxic mold.

Mother Colony. A growth of Stachybotrys or other toxic mold that feeds on a substantial amount of cellulose and a constant water source; often hidden from view inside walls or in other areas.

Multiple Chemical Sensitivity (MCS). A condition in which sufferers respond negatively to a wide variety of chemicals that do not affect most people; may abate with successful avoidance of toxic mold.

Multiple Susceptible (or Multisusceptible) Genotype. HLA DR category that indicates an individual who is unable to easily detoxify a variety of biotoxins from the system.

Multiply Antibiotic Resistant Coagulase Negative Staphylococci (MARCoNS). A bacteria that colonizes the skin and nose of MSH-deficient patients, making their recovery from mold illness more difficult.

Mycotoxin. Poison made by toxic mold.

Mycotoxin Release. Period of time when toxic mold and mycotoxins increase in the outside air; often occurs during weather changes.

Mystery Toxin. A particularly damaging toxin, mostly found outdoors, that seems to be especially associated with sewage.

Nanoparticle. A very small particle of metal that can be produced by mold.

Neurotoxin. Any chemical that has a destructive effect on the brain.

Non-Toxic Mold. Mold that does not manufacture mycotoxins.

Ochratoxin. A mycotoxin that causes kidney disease and that often can be found in coffee, chocolate and other foods.

Off-gas. The process by which toxins or chemicals gradually release from an object into the air.

Perceptify. Determine the presence of toxic mold in an environment or on an object by paying attention to physical, cognitive or emotional responses.

Plume. A moving cloud of toxic mold spores, spore fragments and/or mycotoxins that causes an inside or outside area to be problematic for mold responders.

Potentiated Mycotoxins. Substance made or distributed by toxic mold and incorporating chemicals from the environment.

Power Curve. Extent to which a reactive individual can tolerate additional mycotoxin exposures; being "on top of the curve" provides more resilience.

Pre-contaminated (or pre-molded). A building or item contaminated with toxic mold during the construction, manufacturing or distribution process.

Pristine. Free of a level of mycotoxins or other substances having a negative effect on a particular mold responder.

Rainy Weather Response. The tendency of mold responders to experience negative symptoms just before and during rainy periods.

Raking. Tendency of mold spores to move through the air in search of a location providing the conditions in which growth can occur.

Reactivity. The extent to which an individual suffers negative effects that are more than transitory as a result of exposures to toxic mold.

Reaction. Symptoms that occur as a result of an individual being exposed to mold toxins or other substances.

Regular mold toxins. Mold toxins previously studied by researchers.

Relative Shift. The extent to which one environment is found to be significantly better or worse than another; can only be ascertained insofar as the mold responder is not carrying the response from the previous environment on hair or clothing.

Remediation. The process by which toxic mold is carefully removed from a building, thus making it comparatively safe for the majority of the population; often is not sufficient for tolerance by extreme mold reactors.

Safe Space (or Safe Zone). An area in a living space that is kept as clear of toxic mold as possible.

Satellite Colony. A superficial growth of a toxic mold on an observable surface; suggests the presence of a problematic hidden growth.

Satratoxin. A trichothecene mycotoxin made by Stachybotrys.

Secondary Contamination. The transfer of mold spores and spore fragments from an item that has been exposed to toxic mold to another item.

Secondary Metabolites. The poisons released by toxic molds.

Sensitivity. The extent to which an individual can detect the presence of toxic mold based on physical reactions.

Severe Responder (or Severe Reactor). An individual who experiences negative symptoms as a result of exposure to very small amounts of mycotoxins.

Scamp. A fiberglass trailer made in Minnesota.

Sick Building. A building that has a high level of toxic mold, often accompanied by other problematic chemicals.

Sick Building Design. A building design conducive to the growth of toxic molds and chemical toxicity, characterized by centralized duct systems, sealed windows and high levels of insulation.

Sick Building Syndrome. An environmental illness apparently set off by exposure to toxic mold (often along with toxic bacteria and/or toxic chemicals) in a work or home environment.

Sick Region Syndrome. Area of the country that has high levels of outdoor toxic mold; Lake Tahoe-Truckee and post-hurricane Texas and New Orleans are examples.

Slam. A negative effect of a mold exposure that does not dissipate immediately upon obtaining distance from the item or area and the use of decontamination techniques.

Sourcepoint. A colony of mold that is emitting toxic spores.

Spore. The reproductive component of mold; toxic mold releases dormant spores that carry deadly poisons and that can remain viable for a very long time.

Spore Cloud. A clump of toxic mold spores and spore fragments existing in the air outdoors.

Spore Fragment. A piece of a dormant mold spore, especially one carrying mold toxin.

Spot Plume. The presence of toxic mold (or particularly problematic toxic mold) in just part of a building.

Stachybotrys chartarum. A damaging species of toxic mold.

Stachybotrys. A genus of mold that includes the species Stachybotrys chartarum and Stachybotrys atra; also known as "Stachy."

Suicide Response. A brief but intense desire to kill oneself after experiencing a mold slam; may occur in extreme mold avoiders who otherwise have no suicidal inclinations or ideations.

Suicide Season. The period of time between November and February, when outdoor Mystery Toxin often exerts particularly negative effects on mold responders.

Super Stachy. A toxin that seems associated with Stachybotrys but is unusually damaging in its effects.

Super Toxin. A particularly damaging unidentified environmental substance, believed to be made by a mold or other microorganism.

Tahoe Toxin. Another name for the Mystery Toxin.

Tape Lift. A sample of toxic mold used to identify the species that are present.

Threshold of Discernment. The level at which a particular individual can sense that toxic mold is present in the environment.

Tolerance Testing. Making efforts to see if a building, location or object will trigger any negative effects in a particular individual.

Toxic Dust. Substance present in contaminated homes, comprised of toxic mold spores, spore fragments and household dust carrying mycotoxins.

Toxic Mold. Certain species of mold that produce poisons that have a negative effect on people, animals, bacteria and/or other molds.

Toxicant. A manmade chemical.

Toxin. A chemical made by a living organism that has a damaging effect on the body.

Toxin Release. The phenomenon by which adsorbed mycotoxins are released from objects; often occurs to an accelerated extent as a result of barometric pressure drops from weather changes or altitude increases.

Trichothecenes. Poisonous chemicals made by a variety of toxic molds.

Trigger. A chemical substance that has an effect on a sensitive individual.

Uber Toxin. Another name for Hell Toxin.

Universal Reactor. Individual with especially severe Multiple Chemical Sensitivity, exhibiting negative reactions to a very wide variety of chemical substances.

Unmasking. Spending time in a relatively pristine area, so that the chronic negative effects of toxic mold (or other toxic substances) will begin to manifest themselves in acute symptoms upon exposure.

Upregulate. Physical reaction to exposure to toxic mold (or other substance), triggering inflammation.

Visual Contrast Sensitivity Test (VCS Test). An eye exam that detects the presence of toxins (such as mycotoxins and Lyme toxins) in the brain.

Volatile Organic Compounds (VOC's). Organic compounds that evaporate easily; these account for the mustiness of molds but not their most toxic characteristics.

Water Damaged Building (WDB). A building that has had a water event such as a flood or leak, and thus may have been subject to mold growth.

Water Event. A flood, leak or other water intrusion into a building; should be addressed within 24 hours so that Stachy and other toxic mold does not begin to grow.

Wilderness. An area without man-made buildings; often but not always characterized by low levels of toxic mold.

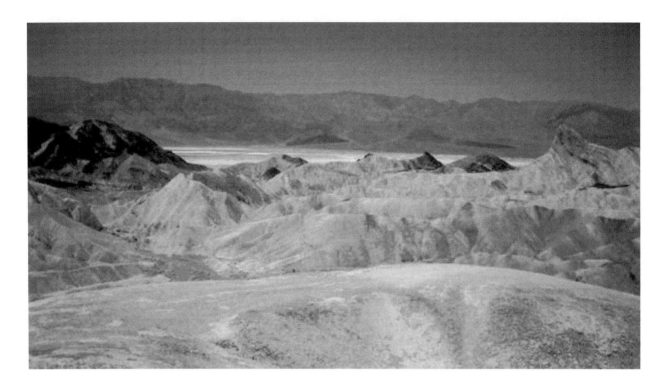

Zabriskie Point at Death Valley National Park in eastern California.

Appendix 3

About the Authors

Lisa Petrison

Lisa Petrison is the executive director of Paradigm Change, an organization that she founded in 2013.

Lisa completed her doctorate in marketing and social psychology at the Kellogg School of Management at Northwestern University in 1998, a few years after first acquiring myalgic encephalomyelitis.

She was a tenure-track professor in the business school at Loyola University Chicago until becoming disabled with the disease in 2001 and mostly bedridden with it in 2007.

Lisa also has served as a marketing consultant and executive speaker for a number of different companies, including California Pizza Kitchen, Wells Fargo, Discover Card, Shell Oil, Hallmark Cards, Visa, Abbott Laboratories, Rodale Press and Cox Cable.

Prior to getting her Ph.D., she worked in marketing/PR for the Chicago Association for Retarded Citizens and in the banking and video games industries, and was a reporter for Adweek magazine.

She has a B.S. in journalism and an M.S. in marketing communications from the Medill School of Journalism at Northwestern University.

Since 2008, Lisa has been focusing her attention on the role of mold toxins and other environmental toxicity in chronic multisystem illness. She and Paul Beith founded the Locations Effect website and Facebook page, focused on the topic of outdoor toxicity in ME/CFS and related illnesses.

Her book about the life of Erik Johnson, *Back from the Edge*, was published in 2013.

Lisa spent about five years traveling around the western half of the US in a non-moldy RV, visiting 25 states and spending time in hundreds of different locations.

She now is mostly recovered (with pre-illness levels of cognitive capacity, resolution of chemical sensitivities and greatly reduced levels of mold reactivities), and credits mold avoidance and detoxification for her improvements.

Her newest venture is "Rabbit Hole," which is designed to provide free information (including books and newsletters) about mold avoidance topics to those who need it.

She currently lives in Taos, NM.

Erik Johnson

Erik Johnson became aware of the negative effects of toxic mold on his health in the early 1970's as a student at Truckee High School in the Lake Tahoe area of California.

He later became very severely ill with the disease that went on to be named chronic fatigue syndrome in the Lake Tahoe epidemic of 1985 (and was one of the first patients to be examined by Dr. Paul Cheney and Dr. Dan Peterson).

He recovered part of his health as a result of mold avoidance in the late 1980's.

Then in 1998, he used the training in bioweapons protocols that he had learned 20 years earlier while serving in the US Army to develop a protocol allowing him to avoid even tiny amounts of mold cross-contamination.

As a result, he went from being extremely sick to climbing Mt. Whitney (the highest mountain in the contiguous US) within six months.

Since then he has continued to work full-time and to exercise vigorously on a regular basis.

Since 2000, he has spent most of his free time helping scientists to understand the role of toxic mold in chronic multisystem illness as well as educating other sufferers with regard to how they can use his techniques to improve their own health.

The book *Back from the Edge* (written by Lisa Petrison) is a summary of Erik's experiences and includes photographs from throughout his life.

A compilation of Erik's public writings from 2000-2010 is available from Paradigm Change under the title *The Role of Toxic Mold in Chronic Fatigue Syndrome*.

Erik also wrote full chapters in Dr. Ritchie Shoemaker's books *Mold Warriors* (Chapter 23, "Mold at Ground Zero for CFS") and *Surviving Mold* (Chapter 17, "The Novice Pilot: CFS and Other Medical Mistakes").

He also is a frequent contributor to the Paradigm Change blog.

Erik currently lives in Reno, Nevada.

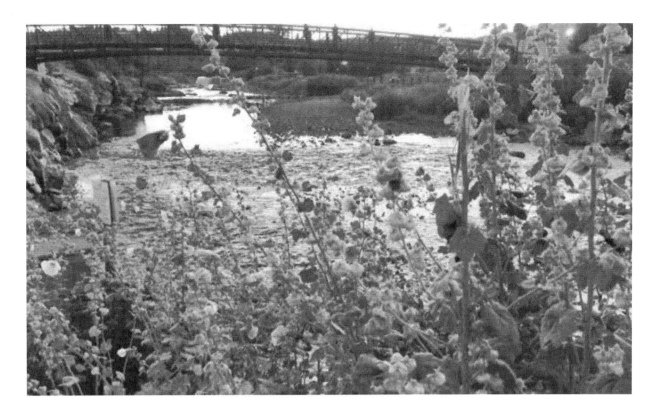

The San Juan River in Pagosa Springs, Colorado.

Appendix 4

Disclaimer & Safety Issues

Following are some extremely important considerations that everyone reading this book should read carefully and then keep in mind.

Disclaimer

Nothing in this book should be taken as any sort of medical advice.

We are not medical practitioners.

Mold avoidance has yet to be studied in any systematic scientific way.

The information in this book is based solely on our own experiences as well as in-depth discussions with other individuals identifying themselves as hyperreactive to toxic mold.

The information in this book is wholly anecdotal and should be taken only as food for thought rather than as providing any definitive direction with regard to a course of action that should be pursued by any particular individual.

Scientific study into this topic of hyperreactivity to toxic mold is desperately needed.

It is our hope that this book will be helpful in making this come about.

Mold Avoidance Safety

Mold avoidance is based on the general principle of removing oneself from exposures to certain kinds of toxic mold and related harmful substances.

Based on the reports of many individuals, it seems that some people cannot tolerate even tiny amounts of these substances without negative effects and therefore may benefit from scrupulous avoidance.

On the surface, it seems that avoiding toxic substances should be a relatively safe approach to addressing any illness.

Anecdotal reports suggest that for the most part this may be the case for mold avoidance, with numerous people who have a hard time tolerating many other treatments reporting benefits from this.

However, one danger reported as being associated with mold avoidance occurs when someone who has successfully gotten clear of problematic toxins for an extended period of time is re-exposed to those toxins.

When that occurs, the acute effect of the toxins can feel worse than when that same person was being chronically exposed without a break.

A typical symptom of people who have gotten relatively clear of these toxins and then been re-exposed is strong suicidal inclination.

Thus, prior to going on a mold avoidance sabbatical, it is essential that people starting mold avoidance consider in advance what they will do if they start to experience substantial mood shifts or suicidal thoughts upon return to the home environment.

A firm plan to move to a different, safer environment if these types of issues emerge is extremely strongly urged before anyone pursues any mold avoidance activities.

Numerous other reactions to problematic substances have been reported from people pursuing mold avoidance.

These have occasionally included passing out, paralysis, inability to speak, seizures or convulsions - symptoms severe enough that hospitalization might be considered appropriate.

However, since few doctors have much knowledge even about mold illness or related illnesses, much less about mold avoidance, unfortunately some emergency rooms may not end up treating individuals suffering from this kind of reaction in appropriate ways.

In addition, certain hospitals have substantial toxic mold problems themselves.

Therefore, especially for people who are very reactive, upfront consideration related to preparing for this kind of circumstance may be a good idea.

Hyperreactivity

The hyperreactivity experienced by people pursuing mold avoidance can alter their lives considerably.

Mold avoiders often have to move to a different location for an extended period or perhaps forever.

Some find it very difficult to find tolerable housing.

They commonly find certain buildings impossible to enter without experiencing negative effects.

When buying new possessions, they may have to be cautious to ensure that items aren't contaminated.

The experience of many mold avoiders is that these difficulties lessen over time, but in general, they often find it difficult to live what most people would consider to be a normal life, at least for a time.

Mold Remediation

Another negative health effect that has occasionally been reported is when individuals misinterpret the concept that "mold is bad" to mean that they should try to clean up the mold in their own living environments.

In some cases, this has resulted in severe, long-term health declines.

Death is a possible outcome of this type of mistake.

No one with chronic multisystem illness should be doing any sort of mold remediation themselves.

While small amounts of these toxins appear to be problematic for many people with this sort of illness, acute exposures to large amounts of the toxins (such as may occur when non-professional remediation is attempted) likely will cause an even greater amount of damage.

Even if the sick person is not present in the home during the process, non-professional remediation has the potential of making a home with a mold problem even more dangerous for people with chronic multisystem illness, since it may allow the spores to spread all over the building rather than remaining relatively contained.

Insofar as any remediation is done, it needs to be conducted in the manner used by competent professionals (for instance, using barriers to seal off the affected areas and removing moldy materials in accordance with hazardous materials protocols).

Another mistake that has the potential of causing harm is when people try to kill hidden mold in their home (for instance, through the use of ozone, dehumidifiers or herbal products such as "Thieves Oil") rather than removing it safely.

The problem is that such measures do nothing about the toxins that are the real problem.

Killing the mold instead has the expected effect of prompting the colonies to release a great deal of dormant toxic spores into the environment all at once, thus increasing the amount of exposure experienced by inhabitants of the building.

Again, especially for people who already are suffering from chronic illness known to be mold-related, any remediation needs to be handled with extreme care using professional techniques -- not with a substance or device available at a local retail store or over the Internet.

The worst of all possible scenarios would be for an ill person to go on a mold avoidance sabbatical to get clear of mold, then return to the problematic home and try to remediate the mold without professional help.

Please don't do this!

Medical Treatment

Mold avoidance is not a substitute for professional medical treatment.

Those who believe that toxic mold may be an issue for them should consult with their healthcare practitioner(s) about their health issues and consider pursuing other treatments that are made available to them, in addition to or as an alternative to pursuing mold avoidance.

Although we discuss medical treatments in Part 6 of this book, it is from the perspective of reporting the experiences that mold avoiders have experienced with them.

This discussion should not be taken as assurance that these treatments will be helpful to any individual or as a recommendation that they be pursued.

It is provided here only as food for thought.

Conclusion

Most importantly, please recognize that mold can be very dangerous.

Mistakes can be extremely costly or deadly.

Therefore, please do not underestimate it and please be safe in dealing with it.

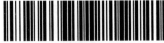
35574270R00173